Workbook for

Laboratory and Diagnostic Testing in Ambulatory Care: A Guide for Health Care Professionals

Third Edition

D1515335

Workbook for

Laboratory and Diagnostic Testing in Ambulatory Care: A Guide for Health Care Professionals

Third Edition

Marti Garrels, MSA, MT (ASCP), CMA (AAMA)
Presently
Medical Assisting Program Consultant
Vancouver, Washington

Formerly
Medical Assisting Program Coordinator
Lake Washington Institute of Technology
Kirkland, Washington

Carol S. Oatis, MSEd, MT SM (ASCP)
Microbiology Adjunct Instructor
Lake Sumter State College
Leesburg, Florida

ELSEVIER
SAUNDERS

3251 Riverport Lane
St. Louis, Missouri 63043

Executive Content Strategist: Jennifer Janson
Senior Content Development Specialist: Jennifer Bertucci
Publishing Services Manager: Hemamalini Rajendrababu
Project Manager: Jayashree Balasubramaniam
Designer: Brian Salisbury

Printed in the United States of America

Last digit is the print number: 10   9   7   6   5   4   3   2

Working together
to grow libraries in
developing countries

www.elsevier.com • www.bookaid.org

Contents

Introduction

This workbook is designed to build mastery over the highly technical and fascinating field of laboratory medicine. Each workbook chapter is organized into five sections: terminology exercises, review questions from basic concepts, procedures, advanced concepts, and check-off procedure sheets for all the procedures presented in the chapter. The completed workbook exercises and check-off procedure sheets fulfill all the competency objectives listed at the beginning of each chapter in the textbook. The appendix of the workbook contains laboratory maintenance logs, report forms, quality control logs, patient logs, a sample health screening assessment form, and a professionalism evaluation form. These forms provide the necessary documentation needed to prove laboratory quality assurance, safety compliance, and proper logging of test results.

TIPS FOR MASTERING EACH CHAPTER

Terminology Exercises

Before reading each chapter, you should become familiar with the technical terms related to the subject. The matching exercises in this workbook can be very helpful for learning the terms, and the Evolve website for students has tutorial drop and drag exercises for mastering terms. Each of the terms is bolded and defined in the context of the chapters to reinforce and build further understanding. There are also powerpoint lectures on the Evolve website for you to fill in the structured notes on your own, or during the classroom lectures.

Basic Concepts, Procedures, Advanced Concepts—Review Questions and Labeling

The questions, pictures, and diagrams in these three sections in the textbook and workbook fulfill the stated objectives for each chapter. The workbook questions are designed to follow the textbook and structured note outline from the Evolve website. You are encouraged to use the textbook alongside the workbook for visual reinforcement and as a reference for finding data from the tables and flow charts. The advanced concepts sections contain more complex critical-thinking exercises as well as referencing detailed laboratory test information in Chapters 3 through 10. Your course instructor may assign one or more of these three sections, depending on the time frame of the course.

Check-off Procedure Sheets

These outcome-based procedure sheets are found at the end of each workbook chapter. You are encouraged to locate the corresponding procedure box in the textbook, which provides pictures of the various steps involved in each procedure. For interested students, video presentations for many of the procedures are also located on the Evolve website. The procedures fall into two categories: *Skill Procedures* (e.g., using a microscope, instructing patients, collecting specimens, staining slides, and performing ECGs and spirometry) and *Analytical Testing Procedures* (e.g., urinalysis, hemoglobin, glucose, HIV and strep tests), in which you follow a test procedure through the preanalytical, analytical, and postanalytical phases to obtain reliable test results. In both cases, it is very important that you read, perform, and check off each step on the sheet as satisfactory or unsatisfactory. The steps marked with an asterisk (*) are critical to demonstrate and pass the competency. The *Skill Procedures* generally are performed with the instructor verifying each step. The *Analytical Testing Procedures* may be performed with a laboratory partner verifying the steps leading up to the test result. The instructor then verifies the final test result and the proper documentation of the test result to fulfill the required measurable outcome.

USING THE WORKBOOK TO SET UP A CLINICAL CLIA-WAIVED LABORATORY

The chapter procedure sheets and all the quality assurance forms provided in the appendix may also be used to set up and monitor a CLIA-Waived Laboratory. The appendix forms are also available electronically on the student Evolve website.

1 Introduction to the Laboratory and Safety Training

INTRODUCTION TO THE LABORATORY—VOCABULARY REVIEW

Match each definition with the correct term.

_____ 1. Most of the population will test within a range of similar results when testing an analyte

_____ 2. Laboratory orders indicating what tests are to be done

_____ 3. A steady state of internal chemical and physical balance

_____ 4. The substance being tested, such as glucose or cholesterol, in a body specimen

_____ 5. A test result indicating a threat to a patient's health

_____ 6. The patient's willingness to follow the treatment plan and take an active role in his or her own health care

_____ 7. Tests that provide simple, unvarying results and require a minimal amount of judgment and interpretation

_____ 8. Clotting ability of blood

_____ 9. A facility or an area within a medical setting in which materials or specimens from the human body are examined or analyzed

_____ 10. The inability to regulate blood sugar levels

_____ 11. Long-lasting, debilitating conditions

_____ 12. Disease-causing microorganisms

_____ 13. Outpatient health care setting in which patients are not bedridden

A. diabetes mellitus
B. homeostasis
C. reference range
D. pathogens
E. compliance
F. CLIA-waived tests
G. chronic disorders
H. analyte
I. critical value
J. ambulatory care
K. requisitions
L. coagulation
M. clinical laboratory

Identify the following acronyms:

14. POCT _____

15. CBC _____

16. POL _____

FUNDAMENTAL CONCEPTS

Overview of the Laboratory

17. List the three reasons a physician would prescribe a laboratory test.

_____

_____

_____

18. List the three ways a specimen is analyzed.

_____

_____

_____

19. List the three types of medical laboratories.

_____

_____

_____

20. List three examples of professional credentials (or titles) obtained by individuals who perform laboratory tests based on their educational degree or certification (see Table 1-1 in the textbook).

Doctorate: 8 or more years of education	Master's: 6 or more years of education	Bachelor's: 4 or more years of education	Associate Degree or Certificate: 1 to 2 years of education

21. Do a self-evaluation of your professionalism by using the form on page 3. Identify two areas you could improve by circling the description "objective" on the left." column.

_____

_____

22. Give three reasons why a physician would want a test performed in the office and three reasons the specimen would be tested at an outside reference or hospital laboratory.

Advantages of In-Office Testing	Advantages of Out-of-Office Testing

23. From the reference laboratory requisition form (see Figure 1-7 in the textbook), write the first three laboratory tests listed in the following categories for blood, and provide the procedure code and blood collection container.

Test Category	Reference Laboratory Tests (see Requisition)	CPT Code (Left of Test)	Container (Right of Test)
Hematology tests			
Chemistry tests			
Serology/immunology tests			

Chapter 1 **Introduction to the Laboratory and Safety Training**

PROFESSIONAL EVALUATION FORM FOR THE LABORATORY CLASSROOM

Student: _____ Date: _____

Class: _____ Semester: _____

Number of Tardies: _____ Number of Hours Absent: _____

Objective	Very Satisfactory 3	Satisfactory 2	Unsatisfactory 1	Comments
Exhibits professional written communication (e.g., appearance, language, grammar)				
Uses the class materials appropriately (e.g., equipment, supplies, computers, cleanup)				
Provides instructor with all necessary information in a timely and organized manner (e.g., meets due dates, make-ups turned in within a week)				
Adheres to specific course policies (e.g., make-up guidelines, skill check-offs, externship guidelines)				
Projects a positive attitude and motivation (e.g., seen during lectures and labs)				
Displays professional verbal communication at all times (e.g., respectful, tactful)				
Maintains confidentiality of all personal interactions at all times (see rules of confidentiality in handbook)				
Projects professional work ethics (e.g., responsible, accountable, independent, full use of laboratory time: practice, study, computer)				
Cooperates with fellow students (e.g., team projects, skill practice, study groups)				
Displays responsible attendance behavior (e.g., arriving on time, calling in if detained or absent, prepared for next class session)				
Dresses appropriately (see handbook)				

Additional Comments: _____

_____

Student Signature _____ Instructor _____

Chapter **1** **Introduction to the Laboratory and Safety Training**

24. Give the metric unit and abbreviation for each basic unit of measurement.

Measurement	Metric Unit	Abbreviation
Weight		
Length		
Volume (capacity)		

25. Give the metric prefix and abbreviation for each of the following.

Fractions	Prefix	Abbreviation
1/10, or 0.1		
1/100, or 0.01		
1/1000, or 0.001		
1/1,000,000, or 0.000001		

26. The following laboratory supplies have temperature storage directions on them. Where should they be stored?

Store at 15° to 30° C _____

Store at 0° C _____

Store at 4° to 8° C _____

27. Give the military times for the following Greenwich times.

3:00 pm _____

8:35 am _____

9:15 pm _____

Noon _____

Chapter **1** **Introduction to the Laboratory and Safety Training**   Copyright © 2015, 2011, 2006 by Saunders, an imprint of Elsevier, Inc. All rights reserved.

SAFETY TRAINING—VOCABULARY REVIEW

Match each definition with the correct term.

_____ 28. A documented plan provided by a facility to eliminate or minimize occupational exposure to bloodborne pathogens

_____ 29. Danger related to the exposure to toxic, unstable, explosive, or flammable materials

_____ 30. A means of transporting an infectious agent or pathogen from the infected individual to another by air, food, hand-to-hand contact, insects, or body fluids

_____ 31. The assumption that the blood or body fluid containing blood from any patient or test kit could be infectious

_____ 32. A disease that is spread within a health care facility

_____ 33. Federal law protecting employees' right to know about the dangers of the hazardous chemicals they may be exposed to under normal working conditions

_____ 34. Through the skin

_____ 35. An area that has been in contact with materials or environmental surfaces where infectious organisms may reside

_____ 36. Specialized clothing or equipment worn by an employee for protection against infectious materials

_____ 37. Efforts and research toward isolating and removing bloodborne pathogens from the workplace

_____ 38. Danger related to exposure to infectious and bloodborne pathogens

_____ 39. Dangers related to electricity, fire, weather emergencies, bomb threats, and accidental injuries

_____ 40. Policies that are recorded, monitored, and evaluated to protect employees from exposure to the pathogens in blood or body fluids

_____ 41. Putting on clothing or equipment as a barrier to a hazard

_____ 42. CDC recommendations for infection control in health facilities

A. chemical hazard
B. Standard Precautions
C. nosocomial infection (HCAI)
D. exposure control plan
E. percutaneous
F. work practice controls
G. Universal Precautions
H. donning personal protective equipment
I. transmission
J. physical hazards
K. engineering controls
L. personal protective equipment
M. hazard communication standard
N. contaminated
O. biohazards

Identify the Following Acronyms

43. Identify the following government safety regulatory agencies by their acronyms:

OSHA _____

HHS _____

CDC _____

FUNDAMENTAL CONCEPTS

Safety Training

44. List three ways that pathogens (infectious organisms) are transmitted.

_____

_____

_____

45. List three methods to sanitize hands. (Hint: Each uses a different cleanser.)

_____

_____

_____

46. Label the following personal protective equipment. (Hint: See Procedure 1-1.)

47. In which of the following disposal containers would contaminated gloves be disposed: wastebasket, biohazard waste container, or biohazard sharps container?

_____

48. List the three major bloodborne pathogens. (Hint: All are viral.)

_____

_____

_____

49. Identify the following acronyms related to infections and to the bloodborne pathogen standard.

HCAIs _____

OPIM _____

PPE _____

PEP _____

50. Identify the following acronyms related to chemical hazard training.

MSDS _____

NFPA _____

HMIS _____

51. List three safety rules that must be observed in the laboratory and explain why.

_____

_____

_____

52. Use the Internet to locate and identify any OSHA or CDC updates on laboratory safety.

_____

Laboratory Safety Checklist

Tour the laboratory with the following safety checklist and perform the bloodborne pathogen training posttest after the tour.

Item	Located
Physical safety	
First-aid kit	
Fire extinguisher	
Evacuation routes	
Fire	
Tornado	
Other (bomb threat)	
Chemical safety items	
Eyewash station	
Material Safety Data Sheets (MSDS)	
Caustic spill kit (if needed)	
Acid spill kit (if needed)	
Hazardous labeling	
Biological safety items	
Bleach disinfectant	
Biohazard spill kit	
Sharps container	
Biohazard container	
Hand sanitizing stations	
Safety devices on needles and lancets	
Personal protective equipment	
Gloves	
Eye goggles and face shields	
Laboratory coat/gown, liquid impenetrable	
Documentation resources	
MSDS/safety manual	
Maintenance logs	
Quality control and patient logs	
Laboratory procedure manual	

1. A laboratory worker exposed to potentially infectious materials on the job may request a vaccine for which blood-borne disease?
   A. HIV
   B. syphilis
   C. hepatitis B
   D. brucellosis

2. Which of the following materials could contain bloodborne pathogens?
   A. bloody saliva
   B. semen
   C. vaginal secretions
   D. all of the above

3. If gloves are worn when cleaning up an accident site, washing the hands afterward is not necessary.
   A. true
   B. false

4. Bloodborne pathogens may enter the system through:
   A. open cuts
   B. skin abrasions
   C. dermatitis
   D. mucous membranes
   E. all of the above

5. All body fluids should be treated as infectious, and direct skin contact with them should be avoided.
   A. true
   B. false

6. Eating, drinking, and smoking should never take place in a laboratory or other area where potential exposure to bloodborne pathogens exists.
   A. true
   B. false

7. What should be done *first* after an exposure incident?
   A. file an exposure report
   B. wash the exposed area
   C. find out if the patient is infected
   D. consult a physician

8. Waste that is dripping blood must be placed in containers that are color coded or clearly labeled "biohazard."
   A. true
   B. false

9. A 10% solution of 1 part household bleach to 9 parts water provides a strong enough solution to decontaminate most surfaces, tools, and equipment effectively if left for 10 minutes.
   A. true
   B. false

10. How can puncture wounds be avoided?
    A. discard used disposable needles in the appropriate container
    B. do *not* recap used needles (use safety activated devices)
    C. practice using safety devices before using on patients
    D. all of the above

Procedure 1-1: Proper Use of Personal Protective Equipment

Person evaluated _____   Date _____

Evaluated by _____   Score _____

Outcome goal	Demonstrate the proper use of personal protective equipment
Conditions	Given the following supplies: 　hand sanitizer 　nonpowdered gloves 　fluid-impenetrable gowns with cuffs at the wrists 　face masks and goggles, or full face shield (if the procedure to be performed has the 　　potential for splashing)
Standards	Required time: 10 minutes Performance time: _____ Total possible points = _____　　Points earned = _____

Evaluation Rubric Codes:
S = Satisfactory, meets standard　　　**U** = Unsatisfactory, fails to meet standard

Preparation	Scores	
	S	**U**
1. Before **donning** (putting on) PPE, remember to perform the hand wash appropriately.		

Procedure	Scores	
	S	**U**
2. Follow the proper sequence for donning PPE.		
a. Put on the gown.		
b. Don any face protectors.		
c. Don disposable nonsterile, nonpowdered, nonlatex, well-fitting gloves.		
d. Extend the gloves over the gown cuffs.		
3. Keep gloved hands away from the face. Remove gloves if they become torn, and perform hand hygiene before donning new gloves. Avoid touching other surfaces and items not involved in the testing process. The outside of the front of the gown is considered contaminated. The "clean" areas of the gown and gloves are on the inside and the back of the gown.		
4. Sequence for removing PPE:		
a. Properly remove gloves as follows:		
Remove one glove by grasping the outside with the other gloved hand and pulling it off.		
Wad up the removed glove in the gloved hand. Slip an ungloved finger under the cuff and fold it over until you can grasp the inside area of the second glove.		
Pull off the second glove inside-out with the first glove still inside.		
b. Remove the face shield.		
c. Remove the gown.		

Follow-up	Scores	
	S	**U**
5. If the gloves have visible blood or body fluid on them, dispose of them in a biohazard waste receptacle.		
6. Perform hand hygiene (hand wash or hand rub) immediately after removing PPE.		
Total Points per Column		

Chapter **1 Introduction to the Laboratory and Safety Training**

2 Regulations, Microscope Setup, and Quality Assurance

VOCABULARY REVIEW

Match each definition with the correct term.

_____ 1. Tests that produce a result measured as a number

_____ 2. A substance or ingredient used in a laboratory test to detect, measure, examine, or produce a reaction

_____ 3. An overall process to aid in improving the reliability, efficiency, and quality of laboratory test results

_____ 4. Materials with known values of the substance measured that help the laboratory achieve accurate and reliable testing by checking if the test system is working

_____ 5. A visible result indicating the presence of a substance a test is designed to detect

_____ 6. Proving competency by testing a specimen from an outside accreditation agency

_____ 7. Tests that look for the presence or absence of a substance

_____ 8. A process in which known samples (controls) are routinely tested to establish the reliability, accuracy, and precision of a specific test system

_____ 9. All components of a test that are packaged together

_____ 10. A built-in positive control to prove the device or test kit is working

_____ 11. The awareness and prevention of both the physical and the procedural risks that may bring about an injury or legal action against the practice

_____ 12. A pattern of narrow and wide bars and spaces; each pattern is encoded with its own particular meaning

_____ 13. When both accuracy and precision are accomplished

_____ 14. Liquid positive and negative controls that are tested the same way as the liquid patient specimen

_____ 15. Ability to produce the same test result each time a test is performed (results are seen clustered together on a target)

_____ 16. The average test result of a series of controls

_____ 17. A statistical term describing the amount of variation from the mean in a dataset

_____ 18. When controls consistently fall within the 2 standard deviations of the mean (results are seen within the center of a target)

_____ 19. Used to plot the daily results of the control samples

_____ 20. A result indicating the absence of the substance that the test is designed to detect

_____ 21. Any substance in a sample, other than the one being measured or detected, whose presence affects the result of the test being performed

_____ 22. When the internal control area on a qualitative test shows no reaction during the testing process

A. reactive/positive
B. quality assurance
C. qualitative
D. quality control
E. kit
F. quantitative
G. reagent
H. proficiency testing
I. controls
J. accuracy
K. Levey-Jennings chart
L. medical office risk management
M. bar codes
N. reliability
O. standard deviation
P. precision
Q. internal control
R. external controls
S. mean
T. invalid test
U. nonreactive/negative
V. interfering substance

Government Acronyms Worksheet

As you write the words for each government acronym or abbreviation, notice its relationship to the various divisions of government and its effect on ambulatory laboratories.

Federal departments	HHS =		CDC =	Department of Labor	
			FDA =		OSHA =
Divisions within the department	OCR = Office of Civil Rights	CMS =			
Laws or regulations affecting laboratories	HIPAA: OCR enforces privacy standards	HIPAA: CMS enforces insurance portability		Infection control:	Infection control, blood:	Hazard communication standard
		CLIA: CMS administers laboratory certifications	CLIA: FDA classifies laboratory test complexity	CDC recommends Standard Precautions for all infectious diseases	OSHA regulates BBPS =	OSHA regulates chemical hazards
Additional acronyms and abbreviations	HIPAA =	CLIA =	CoW =		PPE =	MSDS =
		QA =			OPIM =	HMIS =
	PHI =	QC =	PPM =		PEP =	NFPA =
Additional notes						

CLIA Government Regulations

23. What is the purpose of the Clinical Laboratory Improvement Amendments of 1988 (CLIA 1988) law, and how does it benefit the patient?

_____

_____

24. What are the three categories of testing under CLIA, and under which category is physician-performed microscopy listed?

_____

_____

_____

25. Review Table 2-1 in the textbook, which lists most of the CLIA-waived tests available. Locate three tests in each category, and list their corresponding procedure codes on the following chart:

Test Category	Physician Office Tests	Procedure Code (CPT; 5-digit code)
Hematology tests		
Blood chemistry tests		
Serology/immunology tests		
Microbiology tests (only two)		

26. From the provider-performed microscopy procedure in Table 2-2 in the textbook, write the procedure codes for each of the following:

a. Wet mounts, including preparations of vaginal, cervical, or skin specimens _____

b. Urinalysis (microscopic only) _____

c. All potassium hydroxide preparations _____

27. Label the microscope, and perform the microscopic procedure at the end of the chapter.

28. List the structures under each of the functional areas of the microscope.

Foundational	Illuminating	Magnifying
a.	f.	j.
b.	g.	k.
c.	h.	l.
d.	i.	
e.		

GOOD LABORATORY PRACTICES

Quality Assurance

29. Quality assurance oversees what three areas (or phases) of good laboratory practices? Specimen collection takes place during what phase of good laboratory practices?

_____

_____

_____

30. What is the difference between qualitative tests and quantitative tests, and how does it affect quality control?

_____

_____

_____

31. Explain the relationship of accuracy, precision, and reliability when plotting the results of standard controls.

_____

_____

_____

_____

32. Locate and list the following CDC Tips, Reminders, and Resources from Fig. 2-9 in the textbook:

READY? List four tips to "**Check**" and two tips to "**Perform.**"

Check _____

Check _____

Check _____

Check _____

Perform _____

Perform _____

SET? List a tip to "**Check**" and a tip to "**Wear.**"

Check _____

Wear _____

TEST? List two tips to "**Follow**" and two tips to "**Report.**"

Follow _____

Follow _____

Report _____

Report _____

33. Plot 4 weeks of daily glucose control results on the four blank Levey-Jennings graphs.
    A. Mark the numerical results for each day on the graph.
    B. Identify whether the test system is experiencing a *trend,* a *shift,* a *random error,* or is *out of control.*
    C. How would you correct the quality control issue seen with each week?

    WEEK 1: day 1 = 103, day 2 = 100, day 3 = 98, day 4 = 112, day 5 = 105, day 6 = 99

    A. Week 1 glucose control results show: _____

    B. Possible way to correct: _____

WEEK 2: day 1 = 94, day 2 = 92, day 3 = 93, day 4 = 108, day 5 = 109, day 6 = 107

A. Week 2 glucose control results show: _____

B. Possible way to correct: _____

Chapter **2 Regulations, Microscope Setup, and Quality Assurance**

WEEK 3: day 1 = 90, day 2 = 95, day 3 = 100, day 4 = 105, day 5 = 108, day 6 = 110

A. Week 3 glucose control results show: _____

B. Possible way to correct: _____

WEEK 4: day 1 = 100, day 2 = 103, day 3 = 98, day 4 = 112, day 5 = 115, day 6 = 113

A. Week 4 glucose control results show: _____

B. Possible way to correct: _____

HIPAA Privacy Rule, Risk Management, Electronic Medical Records, and Bar Coding

34. Are laboratory personnel allowed to give an interested party a patient's test results? Why or why not? Base your answer on the Health Insurance Portability and Accountability Act (HIPAA) and risk management principles of avoiding financial and legal consequences.

_____

_____

_____

_____

35. What is the most important use of bar codes in the medical laboratory?

_____

_____

Procedure 2-1: Using a Microscope

Person evaluated _____   Date _____

Evaluated by _____   Score _____

Outcome goal	To bring a stained slide into focus from low power to high dry power and then focus on oil immersion
Conditions	Given a microscope; lens paper; a stained slide; immersion oil; and soft, lint-free tissue
Standards	Time = 15 minutes Accuracy = each step on check sheet is completed, and an image is focused on oil immersion for evaluator check-off before cleanup

Evaluation Rubric Codes:
S = Satisfactory, meets standard   **U** = Unsatisfactory, fails to meet standard

Total possible points = _____   Points earned = _____

NOTE: Steps marked with an asterisk (*) are critical to achieve required competency.

Preparation	Scores	
	S	**U**
1. Carry the microscope with two hands, uncover, and adjust for cleaning.		
- Place one hand under the base, and with the other, grasp the arm of the scope.		
2. Turn the coarse focus until the stage and objectives are farthest apart.		
3. Clean the ocular and all objective lenses with lens paper (clean oil lens last).		
4. Turn the nosepiece to low power (shortest tube).		
- Do not push on objective tubes; use the nosepiece to turn.		
5. Adjust light settings.		
- Bring the condenser all the way up for a stained specimen.		
- Open the iris diaphragm all the way with the lever.		
6. Position a stained slide over the light source.		
- Place the slide with stained side up into the mechanical holder clamp.		
- By using the mechanical control, move the slide until the stained area is above the light.		
7. Adjust the ocular lens to line up with the eyes.		

Procedure	Scores	
	S	**U**
Low-Power Focus		
8. While looking through the oculars, turn the coarse adjustment until color starts to appear, and then turn slowly to bring the image into coarse focus.		
- Always start with the low-power objective to avoid breaking the slide.		
- Move the slide back and forth slightly with the mechanical controls to detect movement.		
9. Move hand to fine-focus adjustment, and turn one way and then the other until the image becomes clear.		
- Make sure both eyes are seeing a clear image; if not, adjust the oculars by turning their individual focus controls.		
10. Move the slide to a place of interest in the center of the visual field, and then turn the nosepiece to high power.		

21

High-Power Focus		
11. Refocus the image by turning the fine adjustment one way and then the other until color is seen; then slowly bring in a clear image.		
- Do not use coarse adjustment because it would make too drastic a change and possibly break the slide. If the fine adjustment cannot focus, go back to low power, and start again with the coarse and fine-focus adjustments.		
- Move the slide so that something interesting is in the middle.		
Oil Immersion Preparation and Focus		
12. Turn the nosepiece halfway between high power and the oil immersion objective.		
13. Place a drop of oil directly on the slide where the condenser light is shining.		
14. Carefully turn the nosepiece until the oil immersion lens dips into the oil and snaps into place.		
*15. While looking into the oculars, move the small fine-focus adjustment back and forth until the image pops into view.		
When image is in view, obtain instructor verification. _____		
- Scan the slide to see cells or organisms.		
- Use one hand on the mechanical control to move the slide, and use the other hand on the fine focus to make continuous adjustments.		

	Scores	
Follow-up: Cleanup and Microscope Maintenance	**S**	**U**
16. Turn off the light, and turn the nosepiece back to the low-power objective.		
- Turn the coarse-focus knob to maximize the distance between the lens and the stage.		
- Remove the slide, and clean the stage with soft, lint-free tissue.		
- Clean oil off the slide with the tissue or xylene.		
17. With lens paper, clean off the ocular lenses and objective lenses; the oil immersion lens is always the last to be cleaned.		
*18. Cover the microscope with a dust-proof cover, and store in a clean, protected area.		
Total Points per Column		

*The instructor or supervisor verifies a successfully focused result. This step is critical to achieve required competency.

2-1

3 Urinalysis

VOCABULARY REVIEW

Match the function with the correct anatomic term.

_____ 1. Functional unit of the kidney

_____ 2. Part of the nephron that contains the glomerulus and glomerular capsule

_____ 3. Structure in the renal corpuscle made up of tangled blood capillaries in which the hydrostatic pressure in the capillaries pushes substances through the capillary pores

_____ 4. Cup-shaped structure surrounding the glomerulus that collects the glomerular filtrate

_____ 5. Urethral opening through which urine is expelled

_____ 6. Slender, muscular tubes 10 to 12 inches long that carry urine formed in the kidneys to the urinary bladder

_____ 7. Hollow, muscular organ that holds urine until it is expelled

_____ 8. Tube that carries urine outside the body

_____ 9. Located behind the peritoneal cavity

_____ 10. Parts of the nephron composed of proximal convoluted tubules, the nephron loop (loop of Henle), and distal convoluted tubules

A. urethral ___ s
B. glomeru___
C. glomerul___ sule
D. urinary bl___
E. renal tubu___
F. nephron
G. renal corpu___
H. ureters
I. retroperitone___
J. urethra

Match each term related to urinalysis with the correct definition (NOTE: Definitions and terms are continued on the next page.).

_____ 11. Caused by treatment or diagnostic procedures

_____ 12. Substance that easily loses electrons

_____ 13. Intact red blood cells in the urine

_____ 14. Protein found in the urine of patients with multiple myeloma

_____ 15. Painful urination

_____ 16. Red cells breaking open and releasing hemoglobin

_____ 17. Expelling of urine, also referred to as voiding and urination

_____ 18. The weight of urine compared with the weight of an equal volume of water; measures the amount of dissolved substances in urine

_____ 19. No urine flow

_____ 20. Sugars (especially glucose) in the urine

_____ 21. To break open

_____ 22. Decreased urine volume

A. electrolyte
B. renal threshold level
C. oliguria
D. bilirubin
E. anuria
F. dysuria
G. nocturia
H. diuresis
I. porphyrin
J. glycosuria
K. reducing substances
L. ketonuria
M. hematuria
N. lyse
O. hemolysis
P. proteinuria
Q. pyuria
R. iatrogenic
S. lipiduria
T. casts

_____ 23. Ketones in the urine

_____ 24. Excessive urination at night

_____ 25. Intermediate substance in the formation of heme (part of hemoglobin)

_____ 26. Element or compound that forms ions when dissolved and is able to conduct electricity

_____ 27. Proteins in the urine

_____ 28. Lipids in the urine

_____ 29. Increase in the volume of urine output

_____ 30. Waste product from the breakdown of hemoglobin

_____ 31. White blood cells in the urine

_____ 32. Elements excreted in the urine in the shape of the renal tubules and ducts

_____ 33. Blood reabsorption limit of a substance and the point at which the substance is then excreted in the urine

_____ 34. Scale that measures the level of acidity or alkalinity of a solution

U. micturition
V. pH
W. specific gravity
X. Bence Jones protein

FUNDAMENTAL CONCEPTS

Anatomy of the Urinary System

35. Label the structures of the urinary system.

36. Label the structures of the kidney.

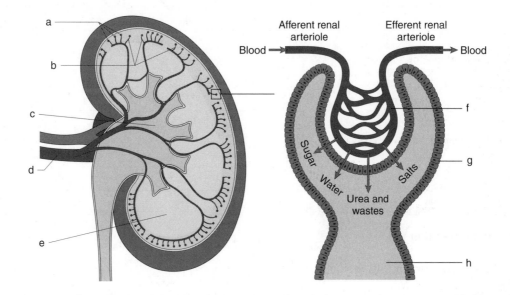

37. List three general functions of the urinary system.

1. _____

2. _____

3. _____

38. Describe the location of the kidneys in the body.

_____

_____

39. List the functions of the nephron.

_____

_____

40. Name the two structural components of the nephron.

_____

_____

41. List and describe the two components of the renal corpuscle.

_____

_____

_____

42. Describe the three steps of urine formation.

_____

_____

_____

43. Explain the term *renal threshold.*

_____

_____

44. Discuss the importance of a urinalysis.

_____

_____

45. Name the three parts of a urinalysis.

_____

_____

_____

Urine Specimen Collection

46. Discuss the advantages of the first morning specimen.

_____

_____

_____

_____

47. Give three general requirements for all types of urine collection methods.

_____

_____

_____

48. Discuss the proper handling and discarding of urine specimens.

_____

_____

49. When educating a female patient about the steps involved in preparing for midstream clean catch urine, why must the patient understand the importance of wiping from front to back?

_____

_____

_____

CLINICAL LABORATORY IMPROVEMENT AMENDMENT (CLIA)–WAIVED URINALYSIS TESTS

Physical Urinalysis

50. Name the tests that are part of the physical urinalysis.

   _____

   _____

51. List the terms used to describe the appearance of urine.

   _____

   _____

52. Give the range of normal color for urine.

   _____

   _____

53. In what condition can urine have a sweet or fruity odor?

   _____

   _____

54. Discuss three abnormal urine colors and their causes.

   _____

   _____

   _____

55. Describe the relevance of the specific gravity test in the urinalysis.

   _____

   _____

Chemical Urinalysis

56. Discuss the difference between qualitative, quantitative, and semiquantitative testing.

   _____

   _____

57. Label the urinalysis chemistry supplies (see Figure 3-10 in the textbook).

A _____ B _____ C _____ D & E _____

58. Name the 10 urinalysis chemistry tests that are most frequently performed.

1. _____   6. _____

2. _____   7. _____

3. _____   8. _____

4. _____   9. _____

5. _____   10. _____

59. Discuss the reasons for the new method that tests for microalbumin.

_____

_____

_____

60. List three conditions that may cause blood to be found in urine.

_____

_____

_____

61. Explain why a first morning urine sample is recommended when testing for nitrites.

_____

_____

62. If the nitrite test is negative, could bacteria be present in the urine?

_____

_____

63. Name a confirmatory test that can be performed when a urine sample is positive for the bilirubin test.

_____

64. Describe the Clinitek instrument, including its advantages and disadvantages.

_____

_____

_____

65. List three guidelines related to urinalysis chemistry reagent strips.

_____

_____

_____

66. Describe the quality control methods available for urinalysis chemistry testing. (Hint: See question 57.)

_____

_____

67. You just ran the Chek-Stix positive control and recorded the results shown on the next page. Look at the expected results table for a positive control, located on the next page, and then circle the analyte that did **not** fall in its control range. Why do you suppose it did not record correctly? (Hint: Look at how the dipstick enters the urine specimen.)
   - Glucose—negative
   - Bilirubin—positive
   - Ketones—positive
   - Specific gravity 1.015
   - Blood large
   - pH 8.5
   - Protein 100 mg/dL
   - Urobilinogen 3 mg/dL
   - Nitrate—positive
   - Leukocytes—moderate

| Test | Expected Results with Bayer Reagent Strips and Tablets | |
	Chek-Stix Positive Control	Chek-Stix Negative Control
Glucose	100-250 mg/dL	Negative
Bilirubin	Positive	Negative
Ketone	Positive	Negative
Specific gravity	1.000-1.015 (adjusted for pH)	1.010-1.025 (adjusted for pH)
Blood	Moderate, large	Negative
pH	≥ 8.0	6.0-7.0
Protein	Trace, 100 mg/dL (SI units: trace, 1.0 g/L)	Negative
Urobilinogen	≥ 2 mg/dL	0.2-1 mg/dL
Nitrite	Positive	Negative
Leukocytes	Trace, moderate	Negative
Microbumintest	Positive (by using 1:3 dilution of Chek-Stix positive control solution)	Negative
Acetest	Positive	Negative
Clinitest	250-750 mg/dL	Negative
Ictotest	Positive	Negative

68. Circle the patient results that are not in the normal reference range. (Note: Normal results would agree with the "Negative Control" chart above.) What would be the probable cause for the abnormal urinalysis physical and chemical results, and what might the physician do next?
   - Dark yellow
   - Cloudy
   - Glucose—negative
   - Ketones—negative
   - Bilirubin—negative
   - Specific gravity 1.025
   - pH 7
   - Blood 2
   - Urobilinogen 0.2
   - Protein—moderate
   - Nitrite—positive
   - Leukocyte—moderate

   _____

   _____

   _____

69. Circle the patient results that are abnormal compared with the urinalysis "normal" reference ranges (shown on the "Negative Control" chart above). What is the probable cause for the abnormal urinalysis chemical results?
   - Glucose 2%
   - Ketones—moderate
   - Bilirubin—negative
   - Specific gravity 1.025
   - pH 6
   - Blood—negative
   - Urobilinogen 0.2
   - Protein—trace
   - Nitrite—negative
   - Leukocyte—negative

   _____

   _____

70. For the standardized urinalysis Kova system for preparation of the microscopic examination, define the terms *sediment* and *supernatant,* and state which of these is used in the microscopic examination of urine.

_____

_____

71. Name the four factors that can lead to cast formation.

_____

_____

_____

_____

72. Name the crystals that resemble envelopes (with an "X" appearance).

_____

_____

73. What part of the microscopic urinalysis can be performed by a medical assistant?

_____

_____

74. Match the pictures of urine cells, casts, and crystals with their microscopic drawings. (See Figures 3-14 through 3-37 in your textbook.)

Cells

Use these terms to identify the following illustrations: red blood cells (RBCs) on high power, squamous epithelial cells on high power, transitional epithelial cells on high power, white blood cells (WBCs) on high power.

_____

_____

_____

_____

Casts

Use these terms to identify the following illustrations: granular casts, hyaline casts, RBC casts, WBC casts.

_____

_____

_____

_____

Crystals and Other Forms

Use these terms to identify the following illustrations: calcium oxalate crystals, *Trichomonas vaginalis*, triple phosphate crystals, yeast.

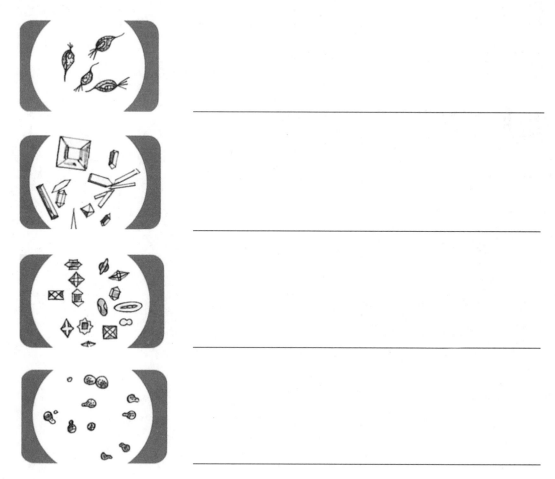

_____

_____

_____

_____

Procedure 3-1: Instructing Patients How to Collect a Clean-Catch Urine Specimen—Female

Person evaluated _____   Date _____

Evaluated by _____

Outcome goal	Instruct a female patient regarding the correct procedure for midstream clean catch specimen.
Conditions	Given the following - Sterile urine collection container and label - Antiseptic towelettes
Standards	Required time: 15 minutes Performance time: _____
Evaluation Rubric Codes: **S** = Satisfactory, meets standard **U** = Unsatisfactory, fails to meet standard Total possible points = _____ Points earned = _____	
NOTE: Steps marked with an asterisk (*) are critical to achieve required competency.	

Preparation	Scores S	Scores U
1. Washed hands and gathered the appropriate equipment.		
2. Greeted and identified the patient.		

Procedure	Scores S	Scores U
3. Instructed patient to sanitize her hands and remove underwear.		
4. Instructed patient to spread apart the labia to expose the urinary opening.		
- Patient told to keep this area spread apart with the nondominant hand during the entire cleaning procedure.		
5. Instructed patient to take one antiseptic towelette and clean one side of the urinary opening from front to back, stressing the importance of the direction.		
- Patient told that cleaning in this direction will prevent anal organisms from being spread to the urinary opening.		
6. Instructed patient to take another antiseptic towelette and clean other side of the urinary opening from front to back, stressing the importance of the direction.		
7. Instructed patient to use a third antiseptic towelette to wipe from front to back directly across the urinary opening, stressing the importance of the direction.		
8. Instructed patient to continue to keep labia spread apart and to urinate a small amount (one third of bladder volume) into the toilet, being careful not to touch the inside of the sterile container.		
- Patient told that the reason for a small amount urinated in the toilet is to flush away micro-organisms that may be around the urinary opening.		
9. Instructed patient to collect the second part of the urine sample into the sterile container.		
- Student was able to state that this would collect the midstream portion of the urine specimen.		
10. Instructed patient to urinate the last portion of the urine into the toilet.		
11. Instructed patient to dry the area with a tissue.		

	Scores	
12. Instructed patient on the correct procedure after the specimen has been collected.		
- Instructed patient to cap the specimen carefully.		
- Instructed patient to place specimen in a certain area after collected in an office setting or to refrigerate if collected at home.		
Follow-up	**S**	**U**
13. After receiving specimen from patient, the sample was labeled correctly, and the requisition was completed if required.		
14. Washed hands.		
*15. Procedure was charted correctly.		
- Charted that female patient was given instructions for midstream clean catch urine collection.		
- Charted reception of specimen from patient.		
Total Points per Column		

Patient Name: _____

Patient Chart Entry: (Include when, what, how, why, any additional information, and the signature of the person charting.)

_____

_____

_____

Procedure 3-1: Instructing Patients How to Collect a Clean-Catch Urine Specimen—Male

Person evaluated _____   Date _____

Evaluated by _____

Outcome goal	Instruct a male patient in the correct procedure for midstream clean catch specimen
Conditions	Given: - Sterile urine collection container and label - Antiseptic towelettes
Standards	Required time: 15 minutes Performance time: _____ Total possible points = _____ Points earned = _____
Evaluation Rubric Codes: **S** = Satisfactory, meets standard **U** = Unsatisfactory, fails to meet standard Total possible points = _____ Points earned = _____	
NOTE: Steps marked with an asterisk (*) are critical to achieve required competency.	

Preparation	Scores	
	S	**U**
1. Washed hands and gathered the appropriate equipment.		
2. Greeted and identified the patient.		

Procedure	Scores	
	S	**U**
3. Instructed patient to sanitize his hands and remove underwear.		
4. If patient is uncircumsized, instructed the patient to retract the foreskin and hold it back during the entire procedure		
5. Instructed the patient to clean the area around the penis opening by starting at the tip of the penis and cleaning downward using a separate antiseptic towelette for each side.		
6. Instructed patient to use a third antiseptic towelette to clean across the opening.		
*7. Instructed patient to urinate a small amount (1/3) into the toilet, being careful not to touch the inside of the sterile container.		
- Patient told that the reason for a small amount urinated in the toilet is to flush away microorganisms that may be around the urinary opening.		
8. Instructed patient to collect the second part of the urine sample into the sterile container.		
- Student was able to state that this would collect the midstream portion of the urine specimen.		
9. Instructed patient to urinate the last portion of the urine into the toilet.		
10. Instructed patient to dry the area with a tissue if needed.		

Follow-up	Scores	
	S	U
11. Instructed the patient on the correct procedure after the specimen has been collected.		
- Instructed the patient to carefully cap the specimen.		
- Instructed patient to place specimen in a certain area after collected in an office setting or to refrigerate if collected at home.		
12. After receiving the specimen from the patient, the sample was labeled correctly and requisition was completed if required.		
13. Washed hands.		
14. Procedure was charted correctly.		
- Charted that male patient was given instructions for midstream clean catch urine collection.		
- Receiving of specimen from patient was charted.		
Total Points per Column		

Patient Name: _____

Patient Chart Entry: (Include when, what, how, why, any additional information, and the signature of the person charting.)

_____

_____

_____

Procedure 3-2: Instructing Patients How to Collect a 24-Hour Urine Specimen

Person evaluated _____ Date _____

Evaluated by _____

Outcome goal	To educate the patient on the correct instructions for collection of a 24-hour urine specimen
Conditions	Given: - Large urine container - Instructions sheet - Requisition
Standards	Required time: 15 minutes Performance time: _____

Evaluation Rubric Codes:
S = Satisfactory, meets standard   **U** = Unsatisfactory, fails to meet standard

Total possible points = _____   Points earned = _____

NOTE: Steps marked with an asterisk (*) are critical to achieve required competency.

Preparation	Scores	
	S	**U**
1. Washed hands and gathered the appropriate equipment.		
2. Greeted and identified the patient.		

Procedure	Scores	
	S	**U**
3. Instructed patient when arising on the first day of the 24-hour collection procedure to empty bladder into the toilet.		
- Instructed patient to record this time.		
4. Instructed the patient that all urine for 24 hours after that first voided specimen must be voided directly into the collection container.		
- Informed the patient to be sure to screw the lid on tightly each time and keep the container refrigerated.		
- Informed the patient that if at any time during the procedure some urine is not collected, the test will need to start again. Gave examples of this.		
5. Instructed the patient that on the second morning of the 24-hour period the patient must arise at the same time as the first day and urinate directly into the container, keeping this sample.		
- Patient was instructed that the first morning specimen on the second day of the 24-hour period is the last sample collected and is the completion of the collection procedure.		
6. Instructed the patient that on the day the procedure is completed the container must be returned to the physician's office or to the laboratory.		

Follow-up	Scores	
	S	U
7. After the patient completed the procedure and returned the container, the patient was asked if any problems occurred during the collection procedure.		
8. Completed a laboratory requisition form for test ordered.		
9. Prepared the specimen to be transported to the laboratory that will perform the testing.		
*10. Charted the instructions and equipment supplied to the patient.		
- When patient returned with specimen, charted that the specimen was sent to the laboratory, documenting all necessary information concerning the specimen.		
Total Points per Column		

Patient Name: _____

Patient Chart Entry: (Include when, what, how, why, any additional information, and the signature of the person charting.)

_____

_____

_____

Procedure 3-3: Manual Chemical Reagent Strip Procedure

Person evaluated _____   Date _____

Evaluated by _____

Outcome goal	Perform a physical and chemical test on an unknown sample according to stated conditions and standards
Conditions	Given: - Reagent strips - Timing device - Reference chart - Requisition
Standards	Required time: 10 minutes Performance time: _____

Evaluation Rubric Codes:
S = Satisfactory, meets standard   **U** = Unsatisfactory, fails to meet standard

Total possible points = _____   Points earned = _____

NOTE: Steps marked with an asterisk (*) are critical to achieve required competency.

Preparation: Preanalytical Phase	Scores	
	S	**U**
A. Test information		
- Kit or instrument method: **Multistix 10 SG**		
- Manufacturer: **Bayer Corporation**		
- Proper storage (e.g., temperature, light): **room temperature, no direct sunlight**		
- Expiration date _____		
- Lot number _____		
- Package insert or test flow chart _____ yes _____ no		
B. Proper specimen		
- Special patient preparation (e.g., fasting, special diet, first morning specimen): **no special preparation**		
- Appropriate container: **clean container without preservatives**		
- Amount of specimen: **25 to 50 mL well-mixed urine**		
C. Personal protective equipment: **gloves, gown, and biohazard container**		

Procedure: Analytical Phase	Scores	
	S	**U**
*D. Performed/observed quality control methods		
1. Semiquantitative liquid controls		
- Control levels: Normal _____ Abnormal _____		

3-3

*E. Performed patient test		
1. Hands were sanitized and equipment assembled.		
2. Urine was poured into a clear container or centrifuge tube.		
3. The color of the urine was determined.		
4. The clarity of the urine was determined.		
5. Strip was removed from the bottle, and the bottle was immediately closed. The pads on the strip were not touched, and the strip was held parallel to the chart.		
6. The pads were completely covered with urine. The pads were not immersed too long, which could cause the reagents to dissolve and leach out into the urine.		
7. After removing the strip from the urine, the strip was tapped against the side of the tube to remove excess urine.		
8. The color of each strip pad was read at a particular time and compared with the reference chart.		

*Accurate Results (see attached forms) Instructor Confirmation _____

Follow-up: Postanalytical Phase	Scores	
	S	U
*F. Proper documentation _____		
1. On control log: _____ yes _____ no		
2. On patient log: _____ yes _____ no		
3. Documentation on patient chart forms on next page		
4. Identified critical values and took appropriate steps to notify physician.		

Analyte Expected Values

Glucose	**Negative**
Bilirubin	**Negative**
Ketone	**Negative**
Specific gravity	**1.005-1.030**
Blood	**Negative**
pH	**6.0-8.0**
Protein	**Negative/trace**
Urobilirubin	**Normal**
Nitrite	**Negative**
Leukocytes	**Negative**

G. Proper disposal and disinfection		
1. Disposed of strip into appropriate biohazard containers.		
2. Poured the remaining urine down sink with stream of water and placed container in appropriate waste container.		
3. Disinfected test area and instruments according to OSHA guidelines.		
4. Sanitized hands after removing gloves.		
Total Points per Column		

Patient Name: _____

Patient Chart Entry: (Include when, what, how, why, any additional information, and the signature of the person charting.)

_____

_____

_____

3-3

Form 1

Patient: ___
Doctor: ___
DOB: ___
Date/Time Spec. Collected: ___
Date/Time Spec. Completed: ___

	TEST	REFERENCE	RESULT	TEST	REFERENCE	RESULT	TEST	REFERENCE	RESULT
☐ VOID	Color	Yellow		Blood	Neg		WBC	0 - 5 HPF	
☐ CC	Char.	Clear		pH	5.0 - 8.0		RBC	0 - 3 HPF	
☐ CATH	Glucose	Neg		Protein	Neg		Epith.	D	
☐ TURBID	Bilirubin	Neg		Urobili	0.2 - 1.0 EU		Cryst.	0 - 3 HPF	
☐ HAZY	Ketone	Neg		Nitrite	Neg				
☐ CLEAR	Sp. Gr	1,000 - 1,030		Leuk	Neg				

MICRO

	TEST	REFERENCE	RESULT
	Bact.	0 - 5	
	Mucus	0	
	Casts	0	

OTHER:

Form 2

Patient: ___
Doctor: ___
DOB: ___
Date/Time Spec. Collected: ___
Date/Time Spec. Completed: ___

	TEST	REFERENCE	RESULT	TEST	REFERENCE	RESULT	TEST	REFERENCE	RESULT
☐ VOID	Color	Yellow		Blood	Neg		WBC	0 - 5 HPF	
☐ CC	Char.	Clear		pH	5.0 - 8.0		RBC	0 - 3 HPF	
☐ CATH	Glucose	Neg		Protein	Neg		Epith.	D	
☐ TURBID	Bilirubin	Neg		Urobili	0.2 - 1.0 EU		Cryst.	0 - 3 HPF	
☐ HAZY	Ketone	Neg		Nitrite	Neg				
☐ CLEAR	Sp. Gr	1,000 - 1,030		Leuk	Neg				

MICRO

	TEST	REFERENCE	RESULT
	Bact.	0 - 5	
	Mucus	0	
	Casts	0	

OTHER:

Form 3

Patient: ___
Doctor: ___
DOB: ___
Date/Time Spec. Collected: ___
Date/Time Spec. Completed: ___

	TEST	REFERENCE	RESULT	TEST	REFERENCE	RESULT	TEST	REFERENCE	RESULT
☐ VOID	Color	Yellow		Blood	Neg		WBC	0 - 5 HPF	
☐ CC	Char.	Clear		pH	5.0 - 8.0		RBC	0 - 3 HPF	
☐ CATH	Glucose	Neg		Protein	Neg		Epith.	D	
☐ TURBID	Bilirubin	Neg		Urobili	0.2 - 1.0 EU		Cryst.	0 - 3 HPF	
☐ HAZY	Ketone	Neg		Nitrite	Neg				
☐ CLEAR	Sp. Gr	1,000 - 1,030		Leuk	Neg				

MICRO

	TEST	REFERENCE	RESULT
	Bact.	0 - 5	
	Mucus	0	
	Casts	0	

OTHER:

Form 1

Patient: _____
Doctor: _____ DOB: _____
Date/Time Spec. Collected: _____
Date/Time Spec. Completed: _____

	TEST	REFERENCE	RESULT	TEST	REFERENCE	RESULT
☐ VOID	Color	Yellow		Blood	Neg	
☐ CC	Char.	Clear		pH	5.0 - 8.0	
☐ CATH	Glucose	Neg		Protein	Neg	
☐ TURBID	Bilirubin	Neg		Urobili	0.2 - 1.0 EU	
☐ HAZY	Ketone	Neg		Nitrite	Neg	
☐ CLEAR	Sp. Gr	1,000 - 1,030		Leuk	Neg	

MICRO	TEST	REFERENCE	RESULT	TEST	REFERENCE	RESULT
	WBC	0 - 5 HPF		Bact.	0 - 5	
	RBC	0 - 3 HPF		Mucus	0	
	Epith.	D		Casts	0	
	Cryst.	0 - 3 HPF				
OTHER:						

Form 2

Patient: _____
Doctor: _____ DOB: _____
Date/Time Spec. Collected: _____
Date/Time Spec. Completed: _____

	TEST	REFERENCE	RESULT	TEST	REFERENCE	RESULT
☐ VOID	Color	Yellow		Blood	Neg	
☐ CC	Char.	Clear		pH	5.0 - 8.0	
☐ CATH	Glucose	Neg		Protein	Neg	
☐ TURBID	Bilirubin	Neg		Urobili	0.2 - 1.0 EU	
☐ HAZY	Ketone	Neg		Nitrite	Neg	
☐ CLEAR	Sp. Gr	1,000 - 1,030		Leuk	Neg	

MICRO	TEST	REFERENCE	RESULT	TEST	REFERENCE	RESULT
	WBC	0 - 5 HPF		Bact.	0 - 5	
	RBC	0 - 3 HPF		Mucus	0	
	Epith.	D		Casts	0	
	Cryst.	0 - 3 HPF				
OTHER:						

Form 3

Patient: _____
Doctor: _____ DOB: _____
Date/Time Spec. Collected: _____
Date/Time Spec. Completed: _____

	TEST	REFERENCE	RESULT	TEST	REFERENCE	RESULT
☐ VOID	Color	Yellow		Blood	Neg	
☐ CC	Char.	Clear		pH	5.0 - 8.0	
☐ CATH	Glucose	Neg		Protein	Neg	
☐ TURBID	Bilirubin	Neg		Urobili	0.2 - 1.0 EU	
☐ HAZY	Ketone	Neg		Nitrite	Neg	
☐ CLEAR	Sp. Gr	1,000 - 1,030		Leuk	Neg	

MICRO	TEST	REFERENCE	RESULT	TEST	REFERENCE	RESULT
	WBC	0 - 5 HPF		Bact.	0 - 5	
	RBC	0 - 3 HPF		Mucus	0	
	Epith.	D		Casts	0	
	Cryst.	0 - 3 HPF				
OTHER:						

Procedure 3-4: Clinitek Analyzer Method for Chemical Reagent Strip

Person evaluated _____ Date _____

Evaluated by _____

Outcome goal	Perform a physical and chemical test on an unknown sample according to stated conditions and standards
Conditions	Given: - Gloves - Multistix 10SG reagent strips or MultistixPro10SL strips - Absorbent paper - Clinitek analyzer
Standards	Required time: 5 minutes Performance time: _____

Evaluation Rubric Codes:

S = Satisfactory, meets standard   **U** = Unsatisfactory, fails to meet standard

Total possible points = _____   Points earned = _____

NOTE: Steps marked with an asterisk (*) are critical to achieve required competency.

Preparation: Preanalytical Phase	Scores	
	S	**U**
A. Test information		
- Kit or instrument method: **Multistix 10 SG and Clinitek instrument**		
- Manufacturer: **Bayer Corporation**		
- Proper storage (e.g., temperature, light): **room temperature, no direct sunlight**		
- Expiration date _____		
- Lot number _____		
- Package insert or test flow chart _____ yes _____ no		
B. Proper specimen		
- Special patient preparation (e.g., fasting, special diet, first morning specimen): **no special preparation**		
- Appropriate container: **clean container without preservatives**		
- Amount of specimen: **25 to 50 mL well-mixed urine**		
C. Personal protective equipment: **gloves, gown, and biohazard container**		
Procedure: Analytical Phase	Scores	
	S	**U**
*D. Performed/observed quality control methods		
1. Semiquantitative liquid controls		
- Control levels: Normal (negative) _____ Abnormal (positive) _____		

*E. Performed patient test		
1. Mixed room-temperature urine sample, and poured it into a conical tube before testing.		
2. Removed strip from bottle, closing bottle immediately. Did not touch the reagent pads.		
3. Followed instructions on the instrument monitor or the manufacturer's flow sheet. ■ Entered technician identification ■ Entered patient information ■ Before pressing the "start" command, had test strip ready to dip into the urine		
4. After pressing start, completed the following within 8 seconds: ■ **Dipped** the strip into the urine, ensuring all the pads were completely covered with urine, but did not immerse it too long ■ **Removed** excess urine from the strip by pulling the nonpad side of the strip along the edge of the container ■ **Blotted** the side of the strip against absorbent paper briefly ■ **Placed** the strip in the Clinitek tray, ensuring it was placed correctly		
5. **Note:** If the reagent strip was placed incorrectly, an error message appeared, and the tray pushed the sample out. The reagent strip was discarded, the instrument was reset, and a new reagent strip was used to run the test again.		
6. While the instrument was measuring timed reagent pads, the color and transparency of the urine specimen were keyed into the analyzer.		
7. When the test was complete, the analyzer displayed and printed the date, the time, the patient's name, the name of the person testing, the results of the 10 tests, the color, and a transparency.		

*Accurate Results (see attached forms or printed form) Instructor Confirmation _____

	Scores	
Follow-up: Postanalytical Phase	**S**	**U**
*F. Proper documentation _____		
1. On control log: _____ yes _____ no		
2. On patient log: _____ yes _____ no		
3. Documentation on patient chart forms on next page		
4. Identified critical values and took appropriate steps to notify physician.		

Analyte Expected Values

Glucose	**Negative**
Bilirubin	**Negative**
Ketone	**Negative**
Specific gravity	**1.005-1.030**
Blood	**Negative**
pH	**6.0-8.0**
Protein	**Negative/trace**
Urobilirubin	**Normal**
Nitrite	**Negative**
Leukocytes	**Negative**

G. Proper disposal and disinfection		
1. Disposed of strip into appropriate biohazard containers.		
2. Disposed of all other regulated medical waste into biohazard bags.		
3. Disinfected test area and instruments according to OSHA guidelines.		
4. Sanitized hands after removing gloves.		
Total Points per Column		

3-4

Patient Name: _____

Patient Chart Entry: (Include when, what, how, why, any additional information, and the signature of the person charting.)

_____

_____

_____

Procedure 3-5: Clinitest Procedure for Reducing Substances Such as Sugars in the Urine

Person evaluated _____ Date _____

Evaluated by _____

Outcome goal	Perform a Clinitest test on an unknown sample
Conditions	Given: - Clinitest bottle of tablets - Clinitest tube - Tube of water with pipette - Urine sample with pipette - Clinitest reference chart
Standards	Required time: 15 minutes Performance time: _____
Evaluation Rubric Codes: **S** = Satisfactory, meets standard **U** = Unsatisfactory, fails to meet standard Total possible points = _____ Points earned = _____	
NOTE: Steps marked with an asterisk (*) are critical to achieve required competency.	

Preparation: Preanalytical Phase	Scores S	U
A. Test information		
- Kit or instrument method: **Clinitest**		
- Manufacturer: **Bayer Corporation**		
- Proper storage (e.g., temperature, light): **room temperature with the lid tightly sealed; protect tablets from light, heat, and moisture**		
- Lot number of kit _____		
- Expiration date _____		
- Package insert available _____ yes _____ no		
B. Specimen information		
- Labeled urine specimen in clean container		
- Amount: **2 or 5 drops (according to directions)**		
C. Personal protective equipment: **gloves, sharps, and biohazard**		
Procedure: Analytical Phase	Scores S	U
D. Performed/observed quality control		
1. Semiquantitative testing controls		
- Control levels: Normal _____ Abnormal _____		

		S	U
E. Performed patient test			
1. Added 5 drops of urine to 10 drops of water in a Clinitest tube.			
2. Tapped the Clinitest tablet into the tube, which was placed in a rack because the boiling reaction that occurs is very hot.			
3. During the boiling reaction, the tube was observed for any color change.			
- The boiling reaction should be observed for the "pass through effect," which results in color change occurring during the reaction and appears negative when the reaction is completed and results are determined.			
4. Shook the tube 15 seconds after the boiling had stopped to mix the contents.			
5. Compared color of the reaction with the Clinitest chart for the 5-drop method and recorded the results.			

*Accurate Results _____ **Instructor Confirmation** _____

Follow-up: Postanalytical Phase	Scores	
	S	**U**
*F. Proper documentation _____		
1. On control log: _____ yes _____ no		
2. On patient log: _____ yes _____ no		
3. Documentation on patient chart (see below)		
4. Identified critical values and took appropriate steps to notify physician. Expected values for analyte: **negative**		
G. Proper disposal and disinfection		
1. Disposed of all other regulated medical waste into biohazard bags.		
2. Disinfected test area and instruments according to OSHA guidelines.		
3. Sanitized hands after removing gloves.		
Total Points per Column		

Patient Name: _____

Patient Chart Entry: (Include when, how, what, why, any additional information, and the signature of the person charting.)

_____

_____

_____

Procedure 3-6: Procedure for the Preparation and the Microscopic Examination of Urine

Person evaluated _____ Date _____

Evaluated by _____

Outcome goal	To prepare a microscopic urinalysis slide, focus the slide on the microscope, and state the elements that can be found under low and high power.
Conditions	Given: - Gloves - Urine specimen - Kova equipment: cap, pipette - Sternheimer-Malbin stain - Test tube - Centrifuge - Microscope
Standards	Required time: 10 minutes Performance time: _____

Evaluation Rubric Codes:
S = Satisfactory, meets standard   **U** = Unsatisfactory, fails to meet standard

Total possible points = _____   Points earned = _____

NOTE: Steps marked with an asterisk (*) are critical to achieve required competency.

Preparation	Scores	
	S	**U**
1. Washed hands, applied gloves, and gathered the appropriate equipment.		
*2. Mixed the correctly identified room-temperature urine specimen.		
*3. Poured the urine sample to the "12 mark" in a urine centrifuge tube and capped the tube.		

Procedure	Scores	
	S	**U**
Performed procedure		
*4. Centrifuged the tube for 5 minutes at 1500 rpm.		
- Stated the definition of sediment and supernatant.		
*5. Carefully removed the spun tube from the centrifuge and removed the cap.		
*6. Carefully placed the Kova pipette into the bottom of the tube.		
- Hooked the clip on the top of the pipette over the outside of the tube.		
*7. Placed index finger on tip of the pipette and decanted off the supernatant by inverting the tube.		
- Stated the approximate amount of sediment that remained in the tube.		

	Scores	
8. Removed the pipette from the tube; added a drop of stain; and reinserted the pipette, squeezing gently to mix the urine sediment and stain.		
- Stated the purpose of using the stain.		
*9. Correctly transferred a drop of the urine sediment to a well in a Kova slide.		
- Did not overfill or underfill the well.		
*10. Allowed the Kova slide to sit for 1 minute.		
- Stated why the slide should sit.		
11. Stated who is qualified to perform a urine microscopic examination.		
12. Demonstrated the ability to focus a slide on the microscope.		
- Focused first with low power with the coarse adjustment.		
- Was able to fine focus with the fine adjustment knob.		
*13. Stated what elements are observed under low power.		
*14. Stated what elements are observed under high power.		

*Accurate Results _____ **Instructor Confirmation** _____

Follow-up: Postanalytical	Scores	
	S	U
Proper disposal and disinfection		
15. Demonstrated the proper procedure for cleaning, carrying, and storing the microscope.		
16. Correctly discarded the equipment in the appropriate containers.		
- Discarded the urine specimen in the appropriate manner.		
17. Removed and discarded gloves in the appropriate biohazard containers.		
18. Sanitized hands.		
19. Demonstrated an understanding of the process for calculating a urinalysis microscopic examination.		
Total Points per Column		

Patient Name: _____

Patient Chart Entry: (Include when, what, how, why, any additional information, and the signature of the person charting.)

_____

_____

_____

4 Blood Collection

VOCABULARY REVIEW

Match each term with the correct definition.

Fundamental Concept Terms

_____ 1. Area in front of the elbow

_____ 2. Blood vessels with a pulse that carry blood away from the heart

_____ 3. Microscopic blood vessels that contain a mixture of arterial and venous blood

_____ 4. Blood collection; derived from the Greek words *phlebo,* meaning vein, and *tomy,* meaning to cut

_____ 5. Blood vessels with valves that carry blood toward the heart

_____ 6. Gently touching and pressing down on an area to feel texture, size, and consistency

_____ 7. Fluid or semifluid substances found in the body

A. humors
B. palpating
C. arteries
D. capillaries
E. phlebotomy
F. veins
G. antecubital space

Blood Collection—Capillary Puncture Terms

_____ 8. All the fluid except blood found in the space between tissues; also referred to as tissue fluid

_____ 9. A newborn child

_____ 10. Inflammation of the bone caused by bacterial infection

_____ 11. Abnormal collection of fluid in interstitial spaces

_____ 12. EDTA

_____ 13. A natural or synthesized chemical that prevents blood from clotting

_____ 14. Skin puncture or "stick" (typically finger stick on adults and heel stick on infants)

_____ 15. Process by which blood flows freely into a capillary tube in microcollection procedures

_____ 16. Condition in which the skin and mucous membranes are blue; caused by an oxygen deficiency

_____ 17. A synthesized anticoagulant that also preserves the blood cells

_____ 18. A natural anticoagulant that prevents the blood from clotting

_____ 19. A test to detect bacteria or organisms growing in the blood

_____ 20. Collecting a small amount of blood

H. capillary action
I. osteomyelitis
J. microcollection
K. interstitial fluid
L. capillary puncture devices
M. lancets
N. blood culture
O. neonate
P. heparin
Q. capillary puncture
R. edema
S. cyanotic
T. anticoagulant

Blood Collection—Venipuncture Terms

_____ 21. Liquid part of whole blood

_____ 22. Removing air to produce a vacuum

_____ 23. Inner tubular space of a needle, vessel, or tube

_____ 24. Immediately

_____ 25. Serum separator tube

_____ 26. Condition in which blood concentration of large molecules such as proteins, cells, and coagulation factors increases

_____ 27. Narrow middle layer of white blood cells and platelets in a centrifuged whole blood specimen

_____ 28. Plasma separator tube

_____ 29. A band placed above the venipuncture site

_____ 30. Liquid part obtained when blood is clotted; lacks the clotting factors

_____ 31. Tubes with air removed to produce a vacuum

A. plasma
B. serum
C. buffy coat
D. evacuated tubes
E. hemoconcentration
F. PST
G. stat
H. evacuated tubes
I. lumen
J. SST
K. tourniquet

Advanced Concepts Terms

_____ 32. Tumor or swelling of blood in the tissues (resulting in bruising during blood collection procedures)

_____ 33. Tiny purple or red skin spots caused by small amounts of blood under the skin; found in patients with coagulation problems; can lead to excessive bleeding during phlebotomy procedures

_____ 34. The breaking open of red blood cells and the release of hemogobin

_____ 35. Fainting

_____ 36. Removal of a breast

L. mastectomy
M. hematoma
N. syncope
O. petechiae
P. hemolysis

FUNDAMENTAL CONCEPTS

37. Explain the differences between arteries, arterioles, capillaries, venules, and veins.

_____

_____

_____

_____

38. Determine if the following substances are higher in the capillary or venous blood.

   a. Hemoglobin _____

   b. Total protein _____

   c. Potassium _____

   d. Glucose _____

   e. Calcium _____

39. Describe the difference in the "feel" between an artery and a vein.

_____

_____

40. Draw a diagram of the most common veins in the antecubital area used for phlebotomy.

41. List the seven items that must be on a laboratory requisition or the patient's electronic record.

a. _____

b. _____

c. _____

d. _____

e. _____

f. _____

g. _____

42. What is the most critical error that a phlebotomist can make before collecting the specimen?

_____

_____

43. Describe the three-way match for patient identification.

_____

_____

44. Explain the proper way to determine a patient's name.

_____

_____

45. Describe and explain the correct positions of a patient when performing phlebotomy.

_____

_____

Capillary Puncture

46. Describe the composition of capillary blood.

_____

_____

_____

47. Label the capillary puncture supplies.

48. List three situations when capillary blood may be used and three situations when this method should not be used.

_____

_____

_____

_____

_____

_____

49. What is the recommended capillary puncture depth for newborns and infants? Explain why.

_____

_____

50. List two types of microtainers that can be used to collect the blood from capillary punctures. (Hint: See Figure 4-6, *C and D,* in the textbook.)

_____

_____

51. List and explain the recommended order of collecting the various colored Microtainers from a capillary puncture.

_____

_____

_____

_____

52. Describe the appropriate capillary puncture collection sites for adults and children and for newborns and infants.

Adults and children: _____

_____

Infants and newborns: _____

_____

53. Why is the first drop of blood wiped away in a capillary puncture?

_____

_____

54. What are the effects of not allowing the alcohol to dry prior to performing the blood collection?

_____

_____

55. What will squeezing the puncture site do to the test results?

_____

_____

56. Describe what to do if the blood stops flowing and not enough blood was obtained.

_____

_____

57. Describe phenylketonuria (PKU).

_____

_____

58. Describe the neonatal screening collection procedure.

_____

_____

_____

_____

59. Discuss the infant age parameters for testing for PKU.

_____

_____

60. In the following case study steps, write **C** if the technique is correct or **I** if the technique is incorrect; explain why in the space provided.

A medical assistant performs a capillary puncture on an adult.

_____ 1. The medical assistant washes his or her hands and puts on gloves.

_____

_____ 2. The site that is chosen is the lateral part of the fingertip (slightly to the side of center) of the middle finger.

_____

_____ 3. The site is cleaned with 30% alcohol.

_____

_____ 4. The puncture is made before the site is dry.

_____

_____ 5. The puncture is made parallel to the whorls of the fingerprint.

_____

61. In the following scenario about a capillary puncture, circle the incorrect techniques. In the space provided, explain the repercussions that could occur from using the incorrect method.

A capillary puncture is performed on the central area of the heel of a newborn infant's foot. The area is cleaned with 70% alcohol; before the alcohol has dried, a puncture is made with a lancet to a depth of 3 mm. Immediately after the puncture, the blood is collected in a capillary tube by squeezing the puncture site. After all the blood has been obtained, pressure is applied to the puncture site, and an adhesive bandage is applied.

_____

_____

_____

_____

_____

62. Explain the difference between serum and plasma, and describe how each is obtained.

_____

_____

63. Label the parts of the Vacutainer system.

64. Place the following tubes in the correct order of draw and name the anticoagulant or additive in each: green, gray, red, lavender.

a. _____; _____

b. _____; _____

c. _____; _____

d. _____; _____

65. Describe how a gel separator tube functions for separating serum and for separating plasma from the cells.

_____

_____

66. Describe the function of the tourniquet. Include the appropriate distance from the puncture site a tourniquet should be placed and the recommended time it should be on the arm.

_____

_____

67. Discuss the criteria for determining whether a tourniquet is on correctly.

_____

_____

68. List the assets and limitations of the topical anesthetic EMLA.

_____

_____

69. Why should the tourniquet be released before removing the needle?

_____

_____

70. Why does the needle need to be held steady during a venipuncture procedure?

_____

_____

71. Name the three methods that can be used to obtain blood from a vein.

_____

_____

_____

72. What are the most frequently used needle lengths and gauges for the Vacutainer system? Which gauge has a larger lumen, 21 or 23?

_____

_____

65

73. List the advantages of using the Vacutainer method.

_____

_____

74. Explain when a butterfly and syringe method would be used.

_____

_____

75. Describe the safety steps of discarding the needle after removing it from the arm with the Vacutainer method.

_____

_____

76. List three conditions that could cause a hematoma.

_____

_____

_____

77. Describe the recommended procedure for transferring blood from a syringe into vacuum tubes.

_____

_____

78. Describe the procedure for determining the appropriate vein for venipuncture.

_____

_____

79. Identify and describe the function of each part of the syringe system.

_____

_____

80. Label the parts of the syringe.

81. Identify and describe the function of each of the components of the butterfly system, including use of the Luer Adapter/Vacutainer method and the syringe method.

_____

_____

82. Label the supplies needed for the butterfly system.

83. Identify two quality assurance steps related to vacuum tube selection. HINT: See Vacutainer Procedure 4-3 Preparation - Pre-analytical text.

_____

_____

84. Discuss the Needle Stick Safety and Prevention Act passed by Congress, which directed the Occupational Safety and Health Administration (OSHA) to revise the bloodborne pathogens standards to require employers to identify and use safer medical devices.

_____

_____

85. In the following case study steps, write **C** if the technique is correct or **I** if the technique is incorrect, and explain why in the space provided.
    A medical assistant is performing a Vacutainer blood collection method.

_____ 1. The patient is told to sit on the end of the examination table.

_____

_____ 2. The medical assistant washes his or her hands, puts on gloves, and then pops the top off of the index finger of the glove.

_____

Chapter **4 Blood Collection**

_____ 3. The tourniquet is applied, and the median cubital vein is determined for use; the tourniquet is then removed.

_____

_____ 4. The chosen site is cleaned with 70% alcohol, working in concentric circles from the inside out, making sure not to backtrack. The tourniquet is then reapplied.

_____

_____ 5. The nondominant hand anchors the vein.

_____

_____ 6. The angle of the needle is 45 degrees as it enters the vein.

_____

_____ 7. After the needle is removed, the safety device is immediately activated.

_____

_____ 8. The needle is unscrewed from the holder and discarded in a sharps container, reusing the holder.

_____

86. In the following scenario about a venipuncture procedure, circle the incorrect techniques. In the space provided, explain the repercussions that could occur from using the incorrect method.

A medical assistant examines an arm to determine the correct vein to use to obtain blood. The arm has very small veins. The medical assistant decides to use the Vacutainer method. The patient's name is determined by asking, "Are you Mrs. Jones?" The patient is then told to sit in a chair with an arm. All the tubes that will be drawn on this patient are prelabeled before the draw. After putting on the tourniquet approximately 3 inches above the puncture site, the arm is cleaned with 70% isopropyl alcohol, starting at the puncture site and moving in a concentric circle outward. The site is retouched by the phlebotomist without cleaning the finger. The needle is inserted into the vein at a 15-degree angle. The lavender tube is filled first, followed by the red tube and gray tube; the green tube is filled last. After the last tube is filled, the needle is removed from the vein, and the tourniquet is removed. Tubes are mixed approximately three times and placed in an upright position in the tray to be taken quickly to the laboratory to perform analytical testing.

_____

_____

_____

_____

_____

_____

_____

68

87. Label all the venipuncture supplies in the figure (see Figure 4-23 in the textbok).

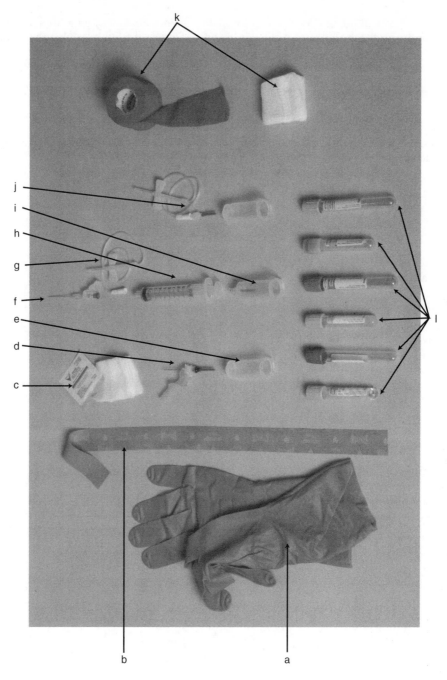

88. Internet activity: Visit one of the following Web sites, and present your findings to the class.

www.mchb.hrsa.gov (Maternal and Child Health Bureau of the Health Resources and Services Administration)

www.aap.org (American Academy of Pediatrics)

www.bd.com (Becton Dickinson)

www.nccls.org (National Committee for Clinical Laboratory Standards)

www.osha.gov (Occupational Safety and Health Administration)

89. The medical assistant is performing a Vacutainer procedure. The needle is inserted into the vein, and the vacuum tube is pushed into the Vacutainer holder. No blood is obtained. Discuss the five possible reasons why this occurred.

_____

_____

_____

90. During a venipuncture procedure, the patient becomes pale, sweats, and hyperventilates. Discuss what occurred and what should be done.

_____

_____

_____

91. The plasma in the vacuum tube appears pink. Explain what this is, list three things that can cause it, and name three tests that can be affected by this condition.

_____

_____

_____

92. After a needle was inserted into a patient's vein, the patient experienced a tingling sensation radiating down the arm. What occurred, and what should the phlebotomist do?

_____

_____

_____

93. If a patient has had a mastectomy, or has a broken arm, or has had an intravenous therapy in the arm on the left side of their body, why would you not draw blood from the left arm in each case?

Mastectomy: _____

Broken arm: _____

Intravenous therapy: _____

94. List five ways to help locate a vein successfully in an obese person.

_____

_____

_____

_____

_____

Procedure 4-1: Capillary Puncture Procedure

Person evaluated _____   Date _____

Evaluated by _____

4-1

Outcome goal	To perform a capillary skin puncture with a retractable, nonreusable lancet
Conditions	Given the following supplies: - Sterile, disposable, retractable, nonreusable lancets (various lengths for the appropriate depth) - Microcollection containers, plastic capillary tubes (with anticoagulant), and sealers - Sterile gauze and 70% isopropyl alcohol pads in sterile packages - Gloves (latex and nonlatex for patients who are allergic) - Biohazard puncture-resistant sharps container - Warming devices, marking pen - Appropriate microcollection containers or testing devices or both depending on what test is ordered
Standards	Required time: 10 minutes Performance time: _____ Total possible points = _____ Points earned = _____

Evaluation Rubric Codes:
S = Satisfactory, meets standard   **U** = Unsatisfactory, fails to meet standard

NOTE: Steps marked with an asterisk (*) are critical to achieve required competency.

Preparation	Scores	
	S	**U**
*1. Identified patient and placed in proper position.		
- Had patient state name.		
- Confirmed identification with patient (birth date or picture ID).		
- Compared with requisition.		
2. Sanitized hands and put on gloves.		
3. Determined the most suitable puncture site and warmed the site.		
- A finger stick: third and fourth finger should be used, making the puncture on the lateral part of the fingertip (slightly to the side of center) and perpendicular to the fingerprint.		
- Newborn or infant (not walking): the medial or lateral plantar section of the foot should be used.		
- Warmed area by massaging the areas five or six times or applied a warmed towel, preemie diaper, or a commercially available device to the site for 3 to 5 minutes.		

Procedure	Scores	
	S	**U**
*4. Disinfected area over chosen site and assembled equipment.		
- Cleaned the site with 70% alcohol.		
- Allowed to dry without fanning or blowing on cleansed site.		
- Assembled the capillary equipment needed, determining the appropriate lancet device to use according to the age and amount of blood needed.		
- Placed all supplies in close proximity to hand.		

Chapter **4** **Blood Collection**

	S	U
5. Pressing hard, made a puncture in the cleaned area at the appropriate site.		
*6. Wiped away the first drop of blood.		
*7. Collected the blood in the proper container by the correct technique.		
- Collected free-flowing drops of blood; did not scoop, scrape, or squeeze the site.		
- If blood was collected in a capillary tube, held the tube horizontal to the site and did not have any air bubbles.		

Follow-up	Scores	
	S	U
8. Asked the patient to apply pressure to site for 3 to 5 minutes.		
9. Gently mixed microcontainers by tilting 8 to 10 times, and labeled all tubes properly.		
- Marked date and time of draw, patient name, and initials or name of phlebotomist.		
- Placed capillary tubes in a vacuum tube, and labeled the vacuum tube.		
*10. Checked site for bleeding, and applied pressure bandage to site.		
- If bleeding continued after 5 minutes, contacted physician.		
- Checked if patient was allergic to bandages before application.		
- Informed parent, if patient is a child, to remove the adhesive bandage after bleeding has stopped because children may choke on it if swallowed.		
11. Determined whether patient was feeling well before dismissing.		
*12. Completed proper documentation on patient chart (see below).		
*13. Properly performed disposal and disinfection.		
- Disposed of all sharps in biohazard sharps containers.		
- Disposed of regulated medical waste in biohazard bags (gloves, gauze).		
- Disinfected test area and instruments according to OSHA guidelines.		
14. Sanitized hands.		
Total Points per Column		

Patient Name: _____

Patient Chart Entry: (Include when, what, how, why, any additional information, and the signature of the person charting.)

_____

_____

_____

Procedure 4-2: Heel Stick for Neonatal Screening Test Procedure

Person evaluated _____ Date _____

Evaluated by _____

Outcome goal	Perform a capillary skin puncture with a retractable, nonreusable lancet
Conditions	Given the following supplies: - Gloves (preferably nonlatex for latex-sensitive patients) - Sterile gauze - Warming device - 70% isopropyl alcohol pads in sterile packages - Sterile, disposable, retractable, nonreusable neonatal lancets with no more than 2-mm depth - Neonatal screening filter paper
Standards	Required time: 15 minutes Performance time: _____ Total possible points = _____ Points earned = _____

Evaluation Rubric Codes:
S = Satisfactory, meets standard   **U** = Unsatisfactory, fails to meet standard

NOTE: Steps marked with an asterisk (*) are critical to achieve required competency.

Preparation	Scores	
	S	**U**
*1. Washed the hands if they were visibly soiled. If not, used an alcohol-based rub for routine decontamination. Applied the hand rub to the palm of one hand and rubbed the hands together, covering all surfaces until dry.		
2. Correctly identified the newborn by using the three-way match, and filled out all the information required on the card.		
3. Applied gloves.		
4. Chose the appropriate site for the heel stick according to the guidelines.		
- Newborn or infant (not walking): the medial or lateral plantar section of the foot should be used.		
- Applied a warmed towel, preemie diaper, or a commercially available device to the site for 3 to 5 minutes.		

Procedure	Scores	
	S	**U**
5. Cleaned the site with 70% isopropyl alcohol. Allowed the alcohol to dry, without fanning or blowing on the site.		
6. With a gloved hand, placed the lancet against the medial or lateral plantar surface of the heel of the foot.		
7. Placed the blade slot area securely against the heel, and firmly and completely depressed the lancet trigger.		
8. Gently wiped away the first drop of blood with sterile gauze or cotton ball.		
9. Applied gentle pressure with the thumb and eased pressure intermittently as drops of blood formed. Applied pressure in such a way that the incision site remained open.		

10. The filter paper should be touched gently against the large blood drop, and in one step, a sufficient quantity of blood should soak through to fill a preprinted circle on the filter paper completely.		
- Do not reapply additional drops in the same circle after leaving the circle.		
- The paper should not be pressed or smeared against the puncture site of the heel.		
- Blood should be applied only to one side of the filter paper, but both sides of the filter paper should be examined to ensure that the blood uniformly saturated the paper.		
11. After all five circles of blood have been collected from the heel of the newborn, the foot should be elevated above the body.		
NOTE: A minimum of three successful circles is needed by the laboratory to test for multiple metabolic disorders.		
12. A sterile gauze pad or cotton swab should be pressed against the puncture site until the bleeding stops.		
- It is not advisable to apply adhesive bandages over skin puncture sites on newborns.		

Follow-up	Scores	
	S	U
13. Logged and charted the procedure.		
14. Allowed filter paper to dry thoroughly on a horizontal, level, nonabsorbent open surface for 3 hours at ambient temperature and away from direct sunlight.		
- Do not touch or smear blood on the filter paper, and do not contaminate the specimen card with cleaning chemicals or other substances.		
- Mailed the thoroughly dried card (Fig. F in textbook Procedure 4-2) in the envelope provided by the health department.		
- Placed capillary tubes in a vacuum tube and labeled the vacuum tube.		
*15. Properly performed disposal and disinfection.		
- Disposed of all sharps in biohazard sharps containers.		
- Disposed of regulated medical waste in biohazard bags (gloves, gauze).		
- Disinfected test area and instruments according to OSHA guidelines.		
16. Sanitized hands.		
Total Points per Column		

Patient Name: _____

Patient Chart Entry: (Include when, what, how, why, any additional information, and the signature of the person charting.)

_____

_____

_____

Procedure 4-3: Vacutainer Method

Person evaluated _____ Date _____

Evaluated by _____

Outcome goal	Perform a venipuncture by the Vacutainer method
Conditions	Given the following supplies: - Disposable gloves - Tourniquet - 70% isopropyl alcohol and sterile gauze pads - Vacutainer double-pointed needle and Vacutainer holder - Correct vacuum tubes for requested tests - Adhesive bandages - Test tube rack - Biohazard sharps containers and bags
Standards	Required time: 10 minutes Performance time: _____ Total possible points = _____ Points earned = _____
Evaluation Rubric Codes: **S** = Satisfactory, meets standard **U** = Unsatisfactory, fails to meet standard	
NOTE: Steps marked with an asterisk (*) are critical to achieve required competency.	

Preparation	Scores	
	S	**U**
*1. Identified and placed patient in proper position.		
- Had patient state name.		
- Confirmed identification with patient (birth date or picture ID).		
- Compared identification with requisition.		
2. Sanitized hands and put on gloves.		
3. Applied tourniquet and determined the most suitable puncture site..		
- Used sufficient pressure to stop venous flow but not arterial flow.		
- Palpated and determined size, depth, and direction of vein.		
4. Removed tourniquet, disinfected area over chosen site, and assembled equipment.		
- Cleansed the site with 70% isopropyl alcohol in concentric circles from inside out.		
- Allowed alcohol to dry without fanning or blowing on cleansed site.		
- Connected the venipuncture assembly in a sterile manner.		
- Placed all supplies in close proximity to arm.		

Procedure	Scores	
	S	**U**
5. Reapplied tourniquet and instructed patient to make a fist (no pumping).		
*6. Disinfected gloved fingers if necessary to palpate site again.		

Chapter **4** **Blood Collection**

	S	U
*7. Uncovered needle, anchored vein, and inserted needle.		
- Pulled skin taut with nondominant thumb 1 to 2 inches below and to the side of the puncture site.		
- Inserted needle ¼ to ½ inch below the vein with bevel up in one swift, continuous motion with dominant hand.		
*8. Pushed tube into needle holder.		
- Used the index and middle fingers of nondominant hand on both sides of the flange and pushed the tube with the thumb of the same hand.		
*9. Followed proper order of draw when filling, removing, and mixing the tubes.		
- Used thumb of nondominant hand against flange and pulled tube out with the fingers of the same hand.		
- Inverted each tube gently to mix blood with additives.		
- Removed the last tube to prevent blood dripping from needle.		
- Instructed patient to release fist.		
*10. Removed tourniquet before taking needle out of arm.		
*11. Placed sterile gauze over needle as it was pulled out and then applied pressure to site.		
- Did not press on gauze until after needle was removed.		
*12. Immediately activated needle safety device and discarded Vacutainer and needle as a unit into the sharps container.		

	Scores	
Follow-up	**S**	**U**
13. Asked the patient to apply pressure to site for 3 to 5 minutes.		
14. Gently mixed tubes by tilting 8 to 10 times, and labeled all tubes properly.		
- Marked patient name, date and time of draw, and initials or name of phlebotomist.		
*15. Checked site for bleeding, and applied pressure bandage to site.		
- If bleeding continued after 5 minutes, contacted physician.		
- Checked if patient was allergic to bandages before application.		
16. Determined if patient was feeling well before dismissing.		
17. Completed proper documentation on patient chart (see below).		
*18. Properly disposed of and disinfected materials.		
- Disposed of all sharps in biohazard sharp containers.		
- Disposed of regulated medical waste (e.g., gloves, gauze) in biohazard bags.		
- Disinfected of test area and instruments according to OSHA guidelines.		
19. Sanitized hands.		
Total Points per Column		

4-3

Patient Name: _____

Patient Chart Entry: (Include when, what, how, why, any additional information, and the signature of the person charting.)

_____

_____

_____

Procedure 4-4: Syringe Method

Person evaluated _____ Date _____

Evaluated by _____

Outcome goal	Perform a venipuncture by the syringe method
Conditions	Given the following supplies: - Disposable gloves - Tourniquet - 70% isopropyl alcohol and sterile gauze pads - Proper-sized syringe and needle - Safety transfer device - Correct vacuum tubes for requested tests - Adhesive bandages - Test tube rack - Biohazard sharps containers and bags
Standards	Required time: 10 minutes Performance time: _____ Total possible points = _____ Points earned = _____
Evaluation Rubric Codes: **S** = Satisfactory, meets standard **U** = Unsatisfactory, fails to meet standard	
NOTE: Steps marked with an asterisk (*) are critical to achieve required competency.	

Preparation	Scores	
	S	**U**
*1. Identified and placed patient in proper position.		
- Had patient state name.		
- Confirmed identification with patient (birth date or picture ID).		
- Compared identification with requisition.		
2. Sanitized hands and put on gloves.		
3. Applied tourniquet and determined the most suitable puncture site.		
- Applied sufficient pressure to stop venous flow but not arterial flow.		
- Palpated and determined size, depth, and direction of vein.		
4. Removed tourniquet, disinfected area over chosen site, and assembled equipment.		
- Cleansed site with 70% isopropyl alcohol in concentric circles from inside out.		
- Allowed alcohol to dry without fanning or blowing on cleansed site.		
- Connected the syringe assembly in a sterile manner.		
- Placed all supplies in close proximity to arm.		

Procedure	Scores	
	S	**U**
*5. Reapplied tourniquet and instructed patient to make a fist (no pumping).		
- Disinfected gloved fingers if necessary to palpate site again.		

	S	U
*6. Removed needle cover, anchored vein, and inserted needle.		
- Pulled skin taut with nondominant thumb 1 to 2 inches below and to the side of the puncture site.		
- Inserted needle ¼ to ½ inch below the vein with bevel up in one swift, continuous motion with dominant hand at the appropriate angle.		
*7. Gently pulled syringe plunger back.		
- Was careful not to pull out of the vein.		
- Instructed patient to release fist.		
*8. Removed tourniquet before taking needle out of arm.		
*9. Placed sterile gauze over needle as it was pulled out, then applied pressure to site.		
- Did not press on the gauze until after the needle was removed.		
*10. Immediately activated syringe needle safety device, unscrewed the needle, and discarded it into the sharps container.		

| | Scores ||
Follow-up	S	U
11. Asked the patient to apply pressure with gauze to site for 3 to 5 minutes.		
12. Filled the vacuum tubes in the proper order of draw by using a transfer safety device.		
- Did not push on the plunger.		
13. Gently mixed tubes by tilting 8 to 10 times, and labeled all tubes properly.		
- Marked patient name, date and time of draw, and initials or name of phlebotomist.		
*14. Checked site for bleeding and applied pressure bandage to site.		
- If bleeding continued after 5 minutes, contacted physician.		
- Checked if patient was allergic to bandages before application.		
15. Determined if patient was feeling well before dismissing.		
16. Completed proper documentation on patient chart (see below).		
*17. Properly disposed of and disinfected materials.		
- Disposed of all sharps, including the transfer device or syringe, in biohazard sharps container.		
- Disposed of regulated medical waste in biohazard bags (gloves, gauze).		
- Disinfected test area and instruments according to OSHA guidelines.		
18. Sanitized hands.		
Total Points per Column		

Patient Name: _____

Patient Chart Entry: (Don't forget to include when, how, what, why, any additional information, and the signature of the person charting.)

_____

_____

_____

Procedure 4-5: Two Butterfly Methods from a Hand and Training Model

Person evaluated _____   Date _____

Evaluated by _____

Outcome goal	Perform a venipuncture by the butterfly method
Conditions	Given the following supplies: - Disposable gloves, tourniquet, 70% isopropyl alcohol, and gauze pads - Winged butterfly set (Safety-Lock or Push Button) with syringe adapter and Vacutainer adapter - Proper-sized syringe or Vacutainer holder - Correct vacuum tubes for requested tests - Adhesive bandages - Test tube rack and biohazard sharps containers and bags
Standards	Required time: 10 minutes Performance time: _____ Total possible points = _____ Points earned = _____
Evaluation Rubric Codes: **S** = Satisfactory, meets standard **U** = Unsatisfactory, failed to meet standard	
NOTE: Steps marked with an asterisk (*) are critical to achieve required competency.	

Preparation	Scores S	Scores U
*1. Identified and placed patient in proper position.		
- Had patient state name.		
- Confirmed identification with patient (birth date or picture ID).		
- Compared identification with requisition.		
2. Sanitized hands and put on gloves.		
3. Applied tourniquet and determined the most suitable puncture site.		
- Applied sufficient pressure to stop venous flow but not arterial flow.		
- Palpated and determined size, depth, and direction of vein.		
4. Removed tourniquet, disinfected area over chosen site, and assembled equipment.		
- Cleansed site with 70% isopropyl alcohol in concentric circles from inside out.		
- Allowed alcohol to dry without fanning or blowing on cleansed site.		
- Straightened out the butterfly tubing.		
- Connected the venipuncture butterfly assembly in a sterile manner to a syringe or a Vacutainer holder.		
- Pushed the plunger back and forth to break the seal if attaching a syringe.		
- Placed all supplies in close proximity to arm or hand.		

Procedure	Scores	
	S	U
*5. Reapplied the tourniquet and disinfected gloved fingers if necessary to palpate site again.		
*6. Removed needle sheath, anchored vein, and inserted needle.		
- Pulled skin taut with nondominant thumb 1 to 2 inches below and to the side of the puncture site.		
- Held the butterfly wings together with the dominant hand and inserted needle ¼ to ½ inch below the vein with bevel up in one swift, continuous motion with dominant hand at the appropriate angle.		
*7. Used the correct technique to obtain blood.		
- Gently pulled syringe plunger back if using syringe method.		
- Used the index and middle fingers of nondominant hand on both sides of the flange and pushed the tube into the holder with the thumb of the same hand if the Vacutainer method was used.		
*8. Tourniquet removed before taking needle out of arm.		
*9. Placed sterile gauze over needle as it was pulled out and then applied pressure to site.		
- Did not press on the gauze until after the needle was removed.		
*10. Immediately activated butterfly needle safety device in a safe manner and disposed of butterfly apparatus properly (illustrations show how to activate the Safety Lock and the Push Button safety devices).		
- If Vacutainer method was used, the butterfly needle, tubing, and Vacutainer holder were discarded in a biohazard sharps container.		
- If a syringe method was used, the syringe was removed from the butterfly tubing, and the butterfly needle and tubing were discarded into a biohazard sharps container.		

Follow-up	Scores	
	S	U
11. Asked the patient to apply pressure with gauze to site for 3 to 5 minutes.		
12. Filled the vacuum tubes in the proper order of draw by using a transfer safety device if syringe method was used.		
- Did not push on plunger; let vacuum fill the tube.		
13. Gently mixed tubes by tilting 8 to 10 times, and labeled all tubes properly.		
- Marked patient name, date and time of draw, and initials or name of phlebotomist.		
*14. Checked site for bleeding and applied pressure bandage to site.		
- If bleeding continued after 5 minutes, contacted physician.		
- Checked if patient was allergic to bandages before application.		
15. Determined if patient was feeling well before dismissing.		
16. Completed proper documentation on patient chart (see below).		
*17. Properly disposed of and disinfected equipment.		
- Disposed of all sharps, including the transfer device and syringe (if syringe method was used), in biohazard sharps containers.		
- Disposed of regulated medical waste (e.g., gloves, gauze) in biohazard bags.		
- Disinfected test area and instruments according to OSHA guidelines.		
18. Sanitized hands.		
Total Points per Column		

Patient Name: _____

Patient Chart Entry: (Include when, what, how, why, any additional information, and the signature of the person charting.)

_____

_____

_____

Vacuum Tube Exercise

Visualize the following picture:

- *Blue* sky is at the top and is the first tube to draw.
- The *red* and *gold* rays of the sun are on the horizon. They both must be drawn *after* the blue but *before* the remaining anticoagulant tubes.
- *Green* grassy hill is located below the sun rays.
- *Lavender* flowers are at the bottom of the hill growing above the rocks.
- *Gray* rocks are at the bottom of the picture because gray is the last tube to draw.

Next, fill in the blank boxes and missing words from Table 4-5 in the textbook. Cut the rows, mix them up, and then place back in order, or cut all the boxes and put them back together like a puzzle.

Colors in Mountain Picture Placed in Order of Draw from Top to Bottom	Tube Descriptions	Additives	Laboratory Uses
_____ sky at the top	"_____" = tube	_____	_____
_____ and _____ rays above the mountain	red topped tubes = "_____" tube; gold topped (or red/gray) = "_____" tube	clot activator in plastic tubes (red *glass* tubes do not have clot activator); _____ and _____	both yield serum commonly used for testing blood; _____
_____ grass on the mountain	light green topped (or green/gray) "_____" tube; dark green "_____" tube	with lithium or sodium (and gel in the PST tubes)	special tests such as _____
_____ flowers at the base of the mountain	"_____" tube	_____	
_____ rocks at the bottom	"_____" tube	_____	_____ testing

5 Hematology

VOCABULARY REVIEW

Match each definition with the correct term.

_____ 1. Large nuclear cell in the bone marrow that fragments its cytoplasm to become platelets

_____ 2. Stem cell that develops into the three kinds of granulocytes

_____ 3. Abnormally shaped

_____ 4. Acid

_____ 5. Alkaline

_____ 6. Also called rubriblasts, which become red blood cells

_____ 7. Attraction

_____ 8. Blood production

_____ 9. Cells and cell fragments that can be viewed under the microscope

_____ 10. Specialists who evaluate the cellular elements of blood microscopically and analytically

_____ 11. Large, engulfing cells in the tissues that come from monocytes

_____ 12. Many-shaped nucleus; also called PMN or seg

_____ 13. Neutrophils, basophils, and eosinophils group

_____ 14. Newly released red blood cells in the blood that still contain some nuclear DNA

_____ 15. Stem cell capable of becoming any of the blood cells

_____ 16. To change and become something different

_____ 17. Variances in red blood cell size

_____ 18. Platelets

_____ 19. Lymphocytes and monocytes group

A. anisocytosis
B. baso
C. differentiate
D. eosin
E. erythroblasts
F. formed elements
G. granulocytes
H. hematologists
I. hematopoiesis
J. hemocytoblast
K. macrophages
L. myeloblast
M. nongranulocytes
N. -phil
O. poikilocytosis
P. polymorphonuclear
Q. reticulocytes
R. thrombocytes
S. megakaryocyte

_____ 20. A critical element in the production of prothrombin

_____ 21. A traveling clot

_____ 22. Abnormal condition of increased red blood cells

_____ 23. Abnormal decrease in white blood cells

_____ 24. Abnormal increase in white blood cells

_____ 25. Abnormal condition of clotting

_____ 26. Condition in which the red blood cell or hemoglobin levels are below normal

_____ 27. Destruction of the red blood cells

_____ 28. Lack of oxygen in the blood

_____ 29. Like stacked chips

_____ 30. Mathematic ratios of the three red blood cell tests (hemoglobin, hematocrit, and red blood cell count)

_____ 31. Ability of blood to maintain the balance of initiating a clotting response to stop bleeding and at the same time prevent the blood from forming an unwanted stationary clot

_____ 32. Two plasma proteins involved in clotting

_____ 33. Percentage of the five kinds of white blood cells

_____ 34. Cancer of the white blood cells

_____ 35. Increase in color (based on hemoglobin concentration)

_____ 36. Process of clotting

A. anemia
B. embolus
C. fibrinogen, prothrombin
D. hemolysis
E. hemostasis
F. hypoxemia
G. leukemia
H. leukocytosis
I. leukopenia
J. hyperchromia
K. red blood cell indices
L. coagulation
M. rouleaux formation
N. thrombosis
O. vitamin K
P. differential count
Q. polychromia

FUNDAMENTAL CONCEPTS

37. Blood collected from a _____ or a _____ may be used for routine hematologic procedures.

38. The anticoagulated Vacutainer tube containing _____ with a _____ top is used for most hematology tests.

39. Match each blood component with its associated characteristic.

_____ basophil

_____ erythrocyte

_____ monocyte

_____ neutrophil

_____ platelet

_____ lymphocyte

_____ eosinophil

A. Able to engulf foreign matter, especially bacteria

B. Increases in number during allergic reactions

C. Can differentiate into a T cell or a B cell

D. Enters the tissues to mediate the inflammatory response

E. Gathers around the site of a damaged blood vessel and releases chemicals to stimulate clot formation

F. Carries oxygen from the lungs to the cells of the body

G. Becomes a macrophage when it leaves the blood to clean up debris in the tissues

40. Label the missing elements of the following hematopoiesis chart (see Figure 5-3 in the textbook).

a _____

b _____

c _____

d _____

e _____

f _____

g _____

h _____

i _____

j _____

Preparation of a Blood Smear

41. A properly done blood smear will have a _____ edge at the thin end of the slide and a section containing well-distributed blood cells in the _____ of the slide.

42. Blood smears are observed under the _____ lens.

43. When identifying cells, what three characteristics should the technician observe? (Hint: The *RBC Atlas* and *WBC Atlas* describe the general characteristics to observe in blood cells.)

_____

_____

Hemostasis

44. Explain the involvement of each of the following as they pertain to hemostasis. (Hint: See Fig. 5-13.)

Blood vessels: _____

Platelets: _____

Clotting factors: _____

Anticoagulants: _____

45. What is the difference between a thrombus and an embolus?

_____

_____

PROCEDURES: CLINICAL LABORATORY IMPROVEMENT AMENDMENT (CLIA)–WAIVED HEMATOLOGY TESTS

Hemoglobin

46. The two main components of hemoglobin are _____ and _____.

47. What is the function of hemoglobin? _____

Hematocrit

48. Match the following average hematocrit percentages to each population, and note the highest to the lowest averages.

_____ Normal average hematocrit for a woman   A. 56%

_____ Normal average hematocrit for a 6-year-old child   B. 42%

_____ Normal average hematocrit for a man   C. 38%

_____ Normal average hematocrit for a newborn   D. 47%

49. If a sample of capillary blood is used for the microhematocrit, the capillary tube must contain a(n) _____.

50. One medical condition in which a low hematocrit value may be found is _____.

51. True or false: Spun hematocrits should be performed in duplicate. _____

52. Label the layers of the spun hematocrit tube.

Erythrocyte Sedimentation Rate

53. What medical conditions can cause an increased erythrocyte sedimentation rate?

_____

_____

54. What technical interferences during testing would cause an increased erythrocyte sedimentation rate?

_____

_____

Prothrombin Time

55. Describe the role of prothrombin in blood coagulation.

_____

_____

56. Explain the major use of the prothrombin time test.

_____

_____

57. Match each test with its reference range.

_____ hemoglobin   A. 36% to 55%

_____ hematocrit   B. 0 to 20 mm/hr

_____ ProTime   C. 12 to 18 g/dL

_____ ESR   D. Approximately 9 to 18 seconds, or 2 to 2.5 INR

58. Label the Hemocue equipment and supplies (see Procedure 5-2 in the textbook).

After approximately 15–45 seconds the result is displayed.

59. Label the SEDIPLAST ESR supplies (see Procedure 5-5 in the textbook).

60. List the seven tests that comprise the complete blood count.

_____

_____

_____

_____

_____

_____

_____

61. What changes in blood cell size are caused by deficiency of vitamin B_{12}? (Hint: Look under "Anemias" in the textbook.)

_____

_____

62. List two conditions in which anisocytosis is found. (Hint: Look under "Anemias" in the textbook.)

_____

_____

63. Match the red blood cell indices to their reference ranges. (Hint: See Table 5-3 ADULTS column, and note the units associated with each test.)

_____ MCV   A. 26 to 34 pg

_____ MCH   B. 31% to 37% or g/dL

_____ MCHC   C. 82 to 98 µm or fL

64. Hypochromic, microcytic red blood cells have a (higher or lower) _____ MCV and (higher or lower) _____ MCHC.

65. Why does anemia or thrombocytopenia develop in patients with leukemia? (Hint: Consider where and how hematopoiesis occurs.)

_____

_____

66. Name one cause of eosinophilia. (Hint: Review granulocyte functions in "Fundamental Concepts.")

_____

_____

67. Name one cause of neutrophilia. (Hint: Review granulocyte functions in "Fundamental Concepts.")

_____

_____

68. Match the cell with its differential reference percentage according to Table 5-4 in your textbook, circle the two cells with the highest percentages, and underline the two cells with the lowest percentages.

____ band	A. 3% to 9%
____ lymphocyte	B. 50% to 65%
____ neutrophil	C. 0% to 7%
____ monocyte	D. 0% to 1%
____ eosinophil	E. 25% to 40%
____ basophil	F. 1% to 3%

Procedure 5-1: Diff Staining Procedure

Person evaluated _____ Date _____

Evaluated by _____

Outcome goal	Demonstrate the proper staining of a blood smear
Conditions	Given the following supplies: - Quick Diff stain: fixative, red eosin dye, blue baso dye - staining rack - water source (bottled or running water) - bibulous paper - personal protective equipment—gown and gloves
Standards	Required time: 10 minutes Performance time: _____ Total possible points = _____ Points earned = _____
Evaluation Rubric Codes:	
S = Satisfactory, meets standard **U** = Unsatisfactory, fails to meet standard	
NOTE: Steps marked with an asterisk (*) are critical to achieve required competency.	

Preparation	Scores	
	S	**U**
1. Put on personal protective equipment (PPE).		

Procedure	Scores	
	S	**U**
2. Dip the slide in fixative three to five times and allow it to dry completely.		
3. Dip the slide into the red eosin dye three to five times.		
4. Let the excess dye run off and blot the rest away with absorbent paper.		
5. Dip the slide into the blue baso dye three to five times.		
6. After the blue dye is blotted away, rinse the slide thoroughly with water on both sides and allow it to air dry. It may also be pressed between two bibulous papers to help remove the water.		

Follow-up	Scores	
	S	**U**
*7. Observe the slide under the oil immersion lens of the microscope. The challenge is to find the WBCs.		
- Refer to the microscope skill sheet 2-1 in Chapter 2 for the proper steps to bring the slide into focus under the oil immersion lens.		
- The cells and platelets will be enlarged 1000 times (100× oil objective times the 10× ocular lens).		
- The slide will show predominantly RBCs with some small platelet clumps throughout.		
- The two most commonly found WBCs are segmented neutrophils and small lymphocytes.		
- See Table 5-1 for assistance in identifying the WBCs.		
Totals Counts per Column		

Patient Name: _____

Patient Chart Entry: (Include when, what, why, any additional information, and the signature of the person charting.)

_____

_____

_____

Procedure 5-2: Hemoglobin: HemoCue Method

Person evaluated _____   Date _____

Evaluated by _____

Outcome goal	To perform FDA-approved hemoglobin waived test following the most current OSHA safety guidelines and applying the correct quality control
Conditions	Given - Control cuvette - Microcuvette testing devices - Liquid controls: high and low - Alcohol, gauze, safety lancets, and bandage
Standards	Required time: 10 minutes Performance time: _____ Total possible points = _____ Points earned = _____
Evaluation Rubric Codes: **S** = Satisfactory, meets standard **U** = Unsatisfactory, fails to meet standard	
NOTE: Steps marked with an asterisk (*) are critical to achieve required competency.	

Preparation: Preanalytical Phase	Scores	
	S	**U**
A. Test information		
- Kit or instrument method: **Hemocue hemoglobin**		
- Manufacturer: **Hemocue**		
- Proper storage (e.g., temperature, light): **cuvettes stored at room temperature**		
- Lot number on cuvette container: _____		
- Expiration date: _____ **opened container is stable for 3 months**		
- Test flow chart _____ yes _____ no		
B. Specimen information		
- Type of specimen: **capillary blood or EDTA tube blood**		
- Testing device: **microcuvette test device**		
C. Personal protective equipment: **gloves, gown, sharps, and biohazard**		
D. Assembled all equipment, sanitized hands, and applied personal protective equipment		
Procedure: Analytical Phase	**Scores**	
	S	**U**
E. Performed/observed quality control		
1. Quantitative testing controls (if testing method does not have internal controls)		
- Calibration check: **used control cuvette for optics check**		
- Control levels: high _____ low _____		

5-2

F. Performed patient test		
1. Followed proper steps (from test flow chart).		
2. Obtained sufficient drop of blood properly.		
- Wiped away first drop and allowed new drop to form.		
3. Filled cuvette completely in one continuous process; did not top off.		
4. Wiped off excess blood on outside of cuvette immediately.		
- Avoided pulling out blood by contacting tip of cuvette.		
5. Visually inspected for air bubbles and loss of blood from cuvette.		
6. Placed filled cuvette into the cuvette holder and pushed holder into the measuring position.		
7. Result displayed after 30 to 60 seconds.		
*Accurate Results _____ Instructor Confirmation _____		

Follow-up: Postanalytical Phase	Scores	
	S	**U**
*G. Proper documentation		
1. On control log _____ yes _____ no		
2. On patient log _____ yes _____ no		
3. Documented on patient chart (see below)		
4. Identified critical values and took appropriate steps to notify physician		

- Hemoglobin expected values:
     Men = 13.0 to 18 g/dL
     Women = 11.0 to 16.0 g/dL
     Infants = 10.0 to 14.0 g/dL
     Children = increase to adult		

H. Proper disposal and disinfection		
1. Disposed of all sharps in biohazard sharps containers.		
2. Disposed of all other regulated medical waste in biohazard bags.		
3. Disinfected test area and instruments according to OSHA guidelines.		
4. Sanitized hands after removing gloves.		
Totals Counts per Column		

Patient Name: _____

Patient Chart Entry: (Include when, what, why, any additional information, and the signature of the person charting.)

_____

_____

_____

5-2

Procedure 5-3: Hematocrit: General Procedure

Person evaluated _____ Date _____

Evaluated by _____

Outcome goal	Perform FDA-approved hematocrit waived test following the most current OSHA safety guidelines and applying the correct quality control
Conditions	Supplies required: - Plastic capillary pipettes with anticoagulant - Sealant clay (e.g., Critoseal) or self-sealing capillary pipettes - Liquid controls: high and low - Gloves, gown, alcohol, gauze, and lancets - Hematocrit centrifuge with built-in reader or variable reader
Standards	Required time: 15 minutes Performance time: _____ Total possible points = _____ Points earned = _____
Evaluation Rubric Codes: **S** = Satisfactory, meets standard　**U** = Unsatisfactory, fails to meet standard	
NOTE: Steps marked with an asterisk (*) are critical to achieve required competency.	

Preparation: Preanalytical Phase	Scores	
	S	**U**
A. Test information		
- Manufacturer: **Adams Readocrit (or other)**		
- Proper storage of pipettes and sealant (e.g., temperature, light): **room temperature**		
- Expiration date (**2 years or 30 days after opened**)		
- Package insert or test flow chart available: _____ yes _____ no		
B. Specimen information		
- Type of specimen: **capillary blood or venous blood in EDTA tube**		
- Specimen testing device: **two capillary tubes filled at least halfway**		
C. Personal protective equipment: **gloves, gown, face shield**		
D. Assembled all equipment, sanitized hands, and applied personal protective equipment		
Procedure: Analytical Phase	**Scores**	
	S	**U**
E. Performed/observed quality control		
1. Quantitative testing controls		
- **HemataCHEK reference control**		
- Control levels: high _____ low _____ normal _____		
F. Perform patient test		
1. Collected two heparin anticoagulated capillary tubes with blood from a finger or an EDTA tube of blood.		
- Held the capillary tube in a horizontal position or slightly tilted down to allow capillary action to pull the blood into the tube, as shown in Figure A in the textbook.		
- Avoided allowing bubbles into specimen, and filled exactly to the line if using a built-in centrifuge scale or at least ½ full if using a variable reader.		

95

	Scores	

2. Collected whole blood into capillary tubes and sealed one end by pressing and turning in sealant, tapped the sealed end, or held presealed tube in vertical position for 15 seconds.

3. Placed the tubes opposite each other with their clay ends toward the outside of the hematocrit centrifuge to create a balanced centrifuge.

4. Locked the cover firmly against the capillary tubes to prevent breaking, and centrifuged for 5 minutes.

5. Used the built-in scale or the variable scales to adjust the total volume (starting where the clay meets the cells and where the plasma meets the air at the top); determined the percentage of the total volume occupied by the red cells based on where they aligned with the plasma on the scale that is being used.

6. Moved slider and sealed end of capillary tube to far left side of reader tray and rotated tube so entire "RED CELL/PLASMA" diagonal interface could be seen.

7. Checked both readings to see if they were within 2% of each other, and recorded the average of the two tubes.

*Accurate Results _____ **Instructor Confirmation** _____

Follow-up: Postanalytical Phase	Scores	
	S	**U**
*G. Proper documentation		

1. On control log _____ yes _____ no

2. On patient log _____ yes _____ no

3. Documented on patient chart (see below)

4. Identified critical values and took appropriate steps to notify physician
   - Hematocrit expected values:
     Men = 42% to 52%
     Women = 36% to 48%
     Infants = 32% to 38%
     Children = increase to adult levels

H. Proper disposal and disinfection		

1. Disposed of all sharps in biohazard sharps containers.

2. Disposed of all other regulated medical waste in biohazard bags.

3. Disinfected test area and instruments according to OSHA guidelines.

4. Sanitized hands after removing gloves.

Totals Counts per Column		

Patient Name: _____

Patient Chart Entry: (Include when, what, why, any additional information, and the signature of the person charting.)

_____

_____

_____

Procedure 5-4: Hematocrit: HemataSTAT Method

Person evaluated _____ Date _____

Evaluated by _____

Outcome goal	To perform FDA-approved hematocrit waived test following the most current OSHA safety guidelines and applying the correct quality control
Conditions	Supplies required: - Plastic capillary pipettes with anticoagulant - Sealant clay (i.e., Critoseal) - Liquid controls: high and low - Gloves, gown, alcohol, gauze, and lancets
Standards	Required time: 15 minutes Performance time: _____ Total possible points = _____ Points earned = _____

Evaluation Rubric Codes:
S = Satisfactory, meets standard   **U** = Unsatisfactory, fails to meet standard

NOTE: Steps marked with an asterisk (*) are critical to achieve required competency.

Preparation: Preanalytical Phase	Scores	
	S	U
A. Test information		
- Kit or instrument method: **HemataSTAT II**		
- Manufacturer: **Separation Technology, Inc. (STI)**		
- Proper storage (e.g., temperature, light): **room temperature**		
- Expiration date **(2 years or 30 days after opened)**		
- Package insert or test flow chart available: _____ yes _____ no		
B. Specimen information		
- Type of specimen: **capillary blood or venous blood in EDTA tube**		
- Specimen testing device: **two capillary tubes filled at least halfway**		
C. Personal protective equipment: **gloves, gown, face shield**		
D. Assembled all equipment, sanitized hands, and applied personal protective equipment.		
Procedure: Analytical Phase	**Scores**	
	S	U
E. Performed/observed quality control		
1. Quantitative testing controls		
- **HemataCHEK reference control**		
- Control levels: high _____ low _____ normal _____		
F. Perform patient test		
1. Followed proper steps (from test flow chart).		
2. Collected whole blood into capillary tubes and sealed one end by pressing and turning in sealant and then tapped the sealed end.		
3. Inserted the sealed end of capillary tube into the HemataSTAT rotor tube holder.		

97

4. Closed centrifuge lid, locked latch, and pressed "RUN" to spin for 60 seconds.		
5. Waited for beeps, then unlocked latch and opened lid.		
6. Moved slider and sealed end of capillary tube to far left side of reader tray and rotated tube so entire "RED CELL/PLASMA" diagonal interface could be seen.		
7. Pressed "ENT" to read tube.		
8. Moved the slider black line to "SEALANT/RED CELL" interface and pressed "ENT."		
9. Moved the slider black line to "RED CELL/PLASMA" interface and pressed "ENT."		
10. Moved slider black line to "PLASMA/AIR" interface and pressed "ENT."		
11. Noted test result.		
12. Repeated steps 4 to 9 with second tube.		
- Result must be within 2% agreement of first reading.		
- Recorded the average of the two readings.		

*Accurate Results _____   **Instructor Confirmation** _____

Follow-up: Postanalytical Phase	Scores	
	S	U
*G. Proper documentation		
1. On control log _____ yes _____ no		
2. On patient log _____ yes _____ no		
3. Documented on patient chart (see below)		
4. Identified critical values and took appropriate steps to notify physician.		

- Hematocrit expected values:
     Men = 42% to 52%
     Women = 36% to 48%
     Infants = 32% to 38%
     Children = increase to adult levels		

H. Proper disposal and disinfection		
1. Disposed of all sharps in biohazard sharps containers.		
2. Disposed of all other regulated medical waste in biohazard bags.		
3. Disinfected test area and instruments according to OSHA guidelines.		
4. Sanitized hands after removing gloves.		
Totals Counts per Column		

Patient Name: _____

Patient Chart Entry: (Include when, what, why, any additional information, and the signature of the person charting.)

_____

_____

_____

Procedure 5-5: ESR: SEDIPLAST System Procedure

Person evaluated _____ Date _____

Evaluated by _____

Outcome goal	To perform FDA-approved ESR waived test following the most current OSHA safety guidelines and applying the correct quality control
Conditions	Supplies needed: - Plastic Westergren pipette graduated from 0 to 200 mm - SEDIPLAST vials with citrate diluent - Westergren rack for holding the pipettes - Disposal transfer pipette - Timer - Gloves, gown, face shield
Standards	Required time: 70 minutes Performance time: _____ Total possible points = _____ Points earned = _____

Evaluation Rubric Codes:
S = Satisfactory, meets standard   **U** = Unsatisfactory, fails to meet standard

NOTE: Steps marked with an asterisk (*) are critical to achieve required competency.

Preparation: Preanalytical Phase	Scores	
	S	**U**
A. Test information		
- Kit or instrument method: **SEDIPLAST**		
- Manufacturer: **Polymedco, Inc.**		
- Proper storage (e.g., temperature, light): **room temperature**		
- Lot number on package: _____		
- Expiration date: _____		
- Package insert or test flow chart available: _____ yes _____ no		
B. Personal protective equipment: **gloves, gown, face shield**		
C. Proper specimen used for test		
- Type of specimen: **fresh EDTA whole blood up to 2 hours or refrigerated blood up to 6 hours**		
- Specimen testing device: **SEDIPLAST vial and pipette**		
D. Assembled all equipment, sanitized hands, and applied personal protective equipment.		
Procedure: Analytical Phase	**Scores**	
	S	**U**
E. Performed/observed quality control methods: not applicable.		
F. Performed patient test		
1. Removed stopper on vial and filled the vial with blood to indicated mark with a disposable transfer pipette (0.8 mL of blood needed).		
2. Replaced vial stopper and inverted vial several times to mix.		
3. Placed vial in SEDIPLAST rack on a level surface free of vibrations and jarring.		

	Scores	
	S	U

4. Pressed the disposable SEDIPLAST pipette gently through the stopper with a twisting motion and continued to press until the pipette rested on the bottom of the vial (the pipette auto-zeros the blood, and any excess flows into the closed reservoir compartment at the top of the pipette).

5. Set the timer for 1 hour, and let specimen stand undisturbed.

6. After 1 hour, read the numeric results of the ESR (used the scale at the top of the pipette to measure the distance from the top of the plasma to the top of the red blood cells).

*Accurate Results _____ **Instructor Confirmation** _____

Follow-up: Postanalytical Phase	Scores	
	S	U
*G. Proper documentation		
1. On patient log _____ yes _____ no		
2. Documented on patient chart (see below).		
3. Identified critical values, and took appropriate steps to notify physician.		

- ESR expected values:
    Men <50 years old = 0 to 15 mm/hr
    Men >50 years old = 0 to 20 mm/hr
    Women <50 years old = 0 to 20 mm/hr
    Women >50 years old = 0 to 30 mm/hr		

H. Proper disposal and disinfection		
1. Disposed of all sharps in biohazard sharps containers.		
2. Disposed of all other regulated medical waste in biohazard bags.		
3. Disinfected test area and instruments according to OSHA guidelines.		
4. Sanitized hands after removing gloves.		
Totals Counts per Column		

Patient Name: _____

Patient Chart Entry: (Include when, what, why, any additional information, and the signature of the person charting.)

_____

_____

_____

Procedure 5-6: ESR: STRECK 30-minute Procedure

Person evaluated _____ Date _____

Evaluated by _____

Outcome goal	To perform FDA-approved ESR waived test following the most current OSHA safety guidelines and applying the correct quality control
Conditions	Supplies needed: - Black Streck citrate tubes and venipuncture supplies - Streck rack - Timer - Personal protective equipment
Standards	Required time: 40 minutes Performance time: _____ Total possible points = _____ Points earned = _____

Evaluation Rubric Codes:
S = Satisfactory, meets standard   **U** = Unsatisfactory, fails to meet standard

NOTE: Steps marked with an asterisk (*) are critical to achieve required competency.

Preparation: Preanalytical Phase	Scores	
	S	**U**
A. Test information		
- Kit or instrument method: **Streck ESR**		
- Manufacturer: STRECK		
- Proper storage (e.g., temperature, light): **room temperature**		
- Lot number on package: _____		
- Expiration date: _____		
- Package insert or test flow chart available: _____ yes_____ no		
B. Personal protective equipment: **gloves, gown, face shield**		
C. Proper specimen used for test		
■ Collect the blood in a black topped STRECK citrate tube making sure to push and hold the tube stopper firmly against the holder.		
■ Position the tube at an angle the allows the blood stream to hit the wall before mixing with the citrate solution to minimize the formation of blood foam.		
■ The blood will stop flowing near the indicated line on the bottom of the STRECK tube's label.		
■ Immediately remove the tube and tilt 8 to 10 times.		
■ (Note: If using a butterfly needle, a waste tube will be needed to clear the air from the tubing.) Blood from an EDTA tube may also be used. It will need to be transferred into the black tube. In both cases, the blood must be mixed immediately after drawing.		

Procedure: Analytical Phase	Scores	
	S	U
D. Allow the liquid controls and the labeled blood specimen to come to room temperature while mixing thoroughly on a rotating blood mixer for 15 minutes.		
E. Performed patient test		
■ Place the ESR vacuum tube in any free position in the ESR-10 Manual Rack with the stopper in the upright position.		
■ Each tube position is marked with a red circle numbered 1 through 10.		
■ Align the tube so that the bottom of the liquid's curved meniscus is in line with the zero position on the measuring scale.		
■ Note: Do not adjust the position of the tube by pulling on the stopper. Allow the tube to settle in an undisturbed, vertical position for 30 minutes.		
■ After 30 minutes, record the numerical value at the top of the column of sedimented erythrocytes. Report the result as mm/hr modified Westergren method.		
*Accurate Results _____ Instructor Confirmation _____		

Follow-up: Postanalytical Phase	Scores	
	S	U
*F. Proper documentation		
1. On patient log _____ yes _____ no		
2. Documented on patient chart (see below).		
3. Identified critical values, and took appropriate steps to notify physician.		
- ESR expected values: Men <50 years old = 0 to 15 mm/hr Men >50 years old = 0 to 20 mm/hr Women <50 years old = 0 to 20 mm/hr Women >50 years old = 0 to 30 mm/hr		
G. Proper disposal and disinfection		
1. Disposed of all sharps in biohazard sharps containers.		
2. Disposed of all other regulated medical waste in biohazard bags.		
3. Disinfected test area and instruments according to OSHA guidelines.		
4. Sanitized hands after removing gloves.		
Totals Counts per Column		

Patient Name: _____

Patient Chart Entry: (Include when, what, why, any additional information, and the signature of the person charting.)

_____

_____

_____

Procedure 5-7: Prothrombin Time INRatio (HemoSense) Method

Person evaluated _____ Date _____

Evaluated by _____

Outcome goal	To perform FDA-approved prothrombin waived test following the most current OSHA safety guidelines and applying correct quality control
Conditions	Supplies needed: - Gloves - Lancet with 21 gauge - Alcohol, gauze, and bandage for capillary puncture site care - INRatio test strips (at room temperature and sealed in foil container until within 10 minutes of testing) - INRatio meter with digital readout screen that guides the operator through the procedure - Biohazard sharps container
Standards	Required time: 10 minutes Performance time: _____ Total possible points = _____ Points earned = _____
Evaluation Rubric Codes: **S** = Satisfactory, meets standard **U** = Unsatisfactory, fails to meet standard	
NOTE: Steps marked with an asterisk (*) are critical to achieve required competency.	

Preparation: Preanalytical Phase	Scores	
	S	U
A. Test information		
- Kit or instrument method: **INRatio**		
- Manufacturer: **HemoSense**		
- Proper storage (e.g., temperature, light): **foil-pouched test strips are refrigerated and must come to room temperature before opening**		
- Expiration date: _____		
- Lot number on strip: _____		
- Package insert or test flow chart available: _____ yes_____ no		
B. Personal protective equipment: **gloves, gown, face shield**		
C. Proper specimen used for test		
- Type of specimen: **finger stick blood from a finger that has been warmed and gently massaged**		
D. Assembled all equipment, sanitized hands, and applied personal protective equipment.		

Procedure: Analytical Phase	Scores	
	S	U
E. Performed/observed quality control		
- Quantitative testing controls		
- Calibration check: **INRatio instrument and strips are precalibrated; no additional calibration is required**		
- Control levels: **Each test cuvette has three channels that run a level I control, a level II control, and the patient test simultaneously.**		

F. Performed patient test		
1. Turned on the INRatio meter by pressing any button; meter was on a level service and was not moved during testing.		
2. After self-test, the meter read "INSERT STRIP."		
3. Opened a test strip foil pouch, and removed the test strip; inserted the strip into the meter with "INRatio" readable at the bottom of the test strip (see Figure B in the textbook).		
4. Checked that the strip code matched the one on the test strip pouch when "STRIP CODE ####" appeared in the display.		
- If it did, pressed the OK key.		
- If it did not, pressed the UP/DOWN button to change the first digit; pressed OK to enter the new digit; repeated for each new digit until the instrument and the strip codes matched and then pressed OK to finalize the code.		
- Meter then read "WARMING UP."		
5. Prepared the finger by warming, disinfecting, and drying thoroughly.		
- *Waited for the beep* and the prompt "APPLY SAMPLE"; green sample light appeared through the test strip sample well.		
6. Incised the finger with the lancet.		
- Wiped away the first drop.		
- Formed a large, hanging drop using gentle continuous pressure.		
7. Applied the hanging drop to the sample well (where the green light shines through the test strip.		
8. Waited while the meter performed the test and calculated the results; message "TESTING SAMPLE" displayed.		
9. The meter beeped, and the results appeared on the display when the test was complete.		
- If an error message occurred, referred to the INRatio User's Guide for proper action.		
10. Read and recorded the INR and PT seconds from the digital screen.		

*Accurate Results INR _____ PT _____ Instructor Confirmation _____

Follow-up: Postanalytical Phase	Scores	
	S	**U**
*G. Proper documentation		
1. On patient log _____ yes _____ no		
2. Documented on patient chart (see below).		

3. Identified critical values and took appropriate steps to notify physician.

ProTime expected values for normal and therapeutic whole blood:

	INR	PT (in seconds)
Normal	0.8-1.2	6.5 to 11.9 seconds for INRatio
Low anticoagulation	1.5-2.0	varies with method used
Moderate anticoagulation	2.0-3.0	varies with method used
High anticoagulation	2.5-4.0	varies with method used

H. Proper disposal and disinfection		
1. Disposed of all sharps in biohazard sharps containers.		
2. Disposed of all other regulated medical waste in biohazard bags.		
3. Disinfected test area and instruments according to OSHA guidelines.		
4. Sanitized hands after removing gloves.		
Totals Counts per Column		

Patient Name: _____

Patient Chart Entry: (Include when, what, why, any additional information, and the signature of the person charting.)

_____

_____

_____

Chapter **5** **Hematology**

6 Chemistry

VOCABULARY REVIEW

Match each definition with the correct term.

_____ 1. Chemicals that produce specific changes in other substances without being changed themselves

_____ 2. Groups of tests providing information on particular organs or body metabolism

_____ 3. Glucose permanently changes the hemoglobin molecule within red blood cells

_____ 4. Abnormal fat levels in the blood

_____ 5. Formation of plaque along the inside walls of blood vessels

_____ 6. Sugars and starches

_____ 7. Sugar in the urine

_____ 8. Cholesterol derived from the diet

_____ 9. Man-made hydrogenated fats

_____ 10. Elevated blood sugar

_____ 11. Fats and proteins that are able to convert to glucose if necessary

_____ 12. Electrolytes consisting of positively or negatively charged particles

_____ 13. Excessively high blood insulin levels

_____ 14. Hormone produced by the pancreas to lower blood glucose

_____ 15. Diagnosis based on the patient's initial signs and symptoms

_____ 16. Excessive fat in blood, giving a milky appearance in the plasma

_____ 17. Condition of excessive ketones in the blood causing an acid condition

_____ 18. Hormone produced by the pancreas to raise blood glucose

_____ 19. Stored form of glucose especially found in muscles and the liver

_____ 20. Cholesterol manufactured in the liver

_____ 21. Final, confirmed diagnosis based on clinical signs and symptoms and the results of diagnostic tests

A. endogenous cholesterol
B. glycogen
C. exogenous cholesterol
D. catalysts
E. hyperinsulinemia
F. glycosylated Hgb
G. hyperlipidemia
H. insulin
I. glucagon
J. trans fats
K. ions
L. glycosuria
M. atherosclerosis
N. panels
O. dyslipidemia
P. carbohydrates
Q. definitive diagnosis
R. hyperglycemia
S. clinical diagnosis
T. ketoacidosis
U. noncarbohydrate energy sources

22. Provide the missing information in the plasma flow chart (see Figure 6-1 in the textbook).

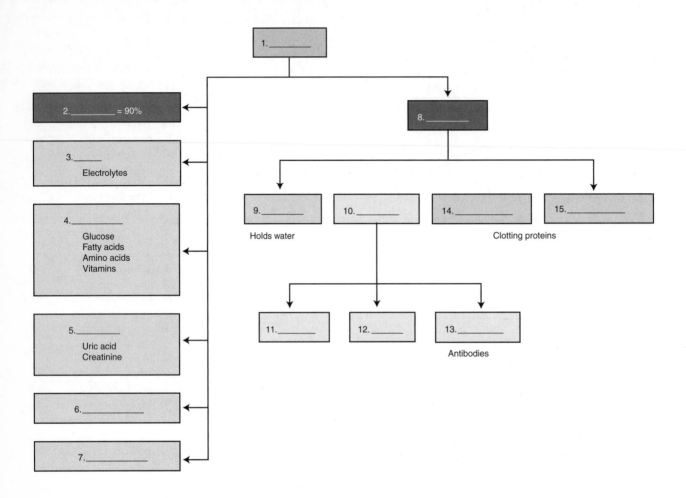

23. Match the categories of chemicals found in plasma with their associated substances (see Figure 6-1 in the textbook).

_____ clotting proteins	A. albumins and globulins
_____ nutrients	B. electrolytes
_____ hormones	C. alpha, beta, and gamma
_____ proteins	D. catalysts
_____ wastes	E. glucose, amino acids, and fatty acids
_____ salts	F. antibodies
_____ gamma globulins	G. thyroid and pituitary glands
_____ enzymes	H. prothrombin and fibrinogen
_____ the three globulins	I. urea, uric acid, creatinine

24. Describe the similarities and differences between the gold "SST" tube and the red "clot" tube.

_____

_____

_____

25. Refer to the sample requisition in the textbook (see Figure 6-4), and identify what tube to use for each of the following tests:

prothrombin time _____   BUN _____

lipid panel _____   CBC w/Diff _____

renal function panel _____   mono test _____

26. When prothrombin and fibrinogen are removed from plasma, the remaining liquid is referred to as

_____.

27. Define the following glucose-related abbreviations.

A_{1c} _____   IGT _____

FBG _____   NIDDM _____

FPG _____   OGTT _____

GTT _____   2-hr PP _____

IDDM _____

28. How is glucose metabolized in the following locations?

Body cells _____

Liver _____

Muscles _____

Adipose tissue _____

29. List the two ways insulin lowers the level of blood glucose.

_____

_____

30. List the two ways glucagon raises the level of blood glucose.

_____

_____

31. What two lifestyle changes can a prediabetic patient make to prevent or delay the development of type 2 diabetes?

_____

_____

32. List three beneficial functions of cholesterol.

_____

_____

_____

33. List the two dietary fats that elevate the bad type of cholesterol (LDL).

_____

_____

34. Define the following lipid-related abbreviations.

HDL _____

LDL _____

TC/HDL ratio _____

VLDL _____

35. List two dietary fats that elevate the good type of cholesterol (HDL).

_____

_____

36. Why is LDL cholesterol referred to as "lousy" cholesterol and HDL referred to as "healthy" cholesterol?

_____

_____

37. Physicians are likely to be more interested in which of the following as a predictive indicator of future myocardial infarction?

    a. Cholesterol value

    b. LDL value

    c. Cholesterol/HDL ratio

    d. HDL value

38. People who exercise regularly, maintain normal weight, and eat mostly unsaturated fats will probably increase their level of

    a. HDL

    b. LDL

    c. Albumin

    d. Glucose

39. When testing for triglycerides, the patient should refrain from alcohol for _____ days before testing and fast for _____ hours before the test.

40. What is the purpose of *calibrating* a blood chemistry analyzer? (Hint: Think of the calibrator checks when running the Cholestech.)

_____

_____

41. Complete the following tasks.
    A. List three reasons or causes why a liquid control would fall outside its designated range.

_____

_____

_____

   B. Using the monthly Levy-Jennings chart at the end of this chapter, record the following control settings and daily results for the normal liquid glucose control (NOTE: On days 13 and 17 the controls were repeated because the first result was out of control.):

   Reference range for control = 96-136 mg/dL

   +2 standard deviations = 136

   +1 standard deviation = 126

   Mean = 116

   −1 standard deviation = 106

   −2 standard deviations = 96

Daily Results

1. 118	7. 108	13. 137	17. repeat 110	23. 120	29. 114
2. 114	8. 114	13. repeat 125	18. 99	24. 114	30. 115
3. 113	9. 120	14. 117	19. 105	25. 133	31. 116
4. 104	10. 118	15. 106	20. 105	26. 123	
5. 101	11. 120	16. 114	21. 110	27. 130	
6. 100	12. 130	17. 94	22. 118	28. 116	

   C. When looking at the chart, were any of the Westgard Rules below broken? (Circle the numbers that apply.)

   Should you continue using the monitor and/or strips? _____
   1. Both levels of control results were outside the manufacturer's reference range (if running a normal and high control). *Note:* This rule does not apply because we are monitoring only one control.
   2. The same control level fell outside of the reference range in two successive runs.
   3. One of the controls fell outside of the plus or minus 1 standard deviation in four successive runs.
   4. One of the controls consistently fell above the mean value or consistently fell below the mean value for 10 consecutive runs.

   D. (OPTIONAL) If available, chart the class results for the liquid glucose control on the Levy-Jennings chart found in the workbook Appendix, and analyze the results based on the Westgard Rules.

42. List three foods that the patient should avoid 2 days before collecting a fecal specimen used for the occult blood test. What is the name of the fecal occult test that does not require eliminating these foods?

_____

_____

_____

43. What is the name of the home fecal occult blood test for which the patient places the test paper directly into the toilet? _____ If the test area of the paper turns green or blue, is the result positive or negative? _____

44. Label the supplies and equipment for the test kit method for A_{1c} (see Procedure 6-2 in the textbook). What is the supply item that must be used for all 20 tests in the kit? _____ May that item be used with cartridges from another kit? _____

45. Label the Cholestech LDX equipment and supplies (see Procedure 6-3 in the textbook).

46. Label the ColoScreen III equipment and supplies (see Procedure 6-4 in the textbook).

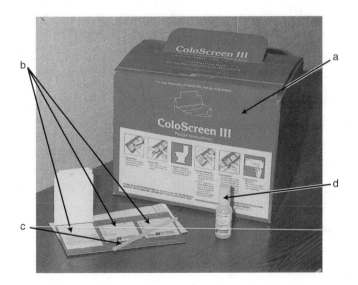

ADVANCED CONCEPTS

Match each procedural and advanced term with the correct definition.

_____ 47. cation

_____ 48. galvanometer

_____ 49. reflectance photometry

_____ 50. troponins I and T

_____ 51. bilirubin

_____ 52. absorbance photometry

_____ 53. anion

_____ 54. i-STAT and Piccolo

_____ 55. transmittance photometry

_____ 56. calibration

_____ 57. occult

_____ 58. gout

_____ 59. myoglobin

A. Form of arthritis caused by accumulation of uric acid crystals in the synovial fluid

B. Hidden or not visible to the naked eye

C. Heme-containing, oxygen-binding protein found in muscles

D. Positively charged ion

E. "Optics check" or setting to ensure the analyzer's optics are working correctly with the testing devices

F. Measurement of the amount of light passing through the solution

G. CLIA-waived chemistry analyzers

H. Heart-specific indicators of a recent myocardial infarction

I. Measurement of the light that reflects off of the specimen

J. Measurement of the amount of light the solution absorbs

K. Waste product from the breakdown of hemoglobin

L. Negatively charged ion

M. Instrument capable of measuring the intensity of light

60. List eight critical chemistry tests that are typically monitored during a medical emergency:

_____   _____

_____   _____

_____   _____

_____   _____

61. Match each of the chemistry panels with their representative group of tests.

_____ cardiac panel

_____ hepatic panel

_____ renal panel

_____ lipid panel

_____ thyroid panel

_____ metabolic panel

_____ electrolyte panel

A. Twelve or more tests

B. BUN, creatinine, uric acid

C. Sodium, potassium, chloride

D. Bilirubin, AST, ALT, ALP, LD, GGT

E. Troponins I and T, CK, LD, ALT, myoglobin

F. TSH, T_4, T_3 uptake

G. TC, HDL, LDL, triglycerides

62. Match the analytes with the medical condition or organ that is being monitored.

_____ uric acid

_____ cholesterol

_____ BUN

_____ glucose

_____ bilirubin

A. Diabetes

B. Hepatitis or liver function

C. Gout

D. Coronary artery disease and atherosclerosis

E. Nephritis or kidney function

Chemistry Abbreviations

63. Using the alphabetical list of abbreviations at the beginning of Chapter 6 in the textbook, identify the six enzyme abbreviations routinely tested for tissue or organ damage. (Hint: Remember enzymes have the suffix -*ase*.) Then identify two organs or the diseases that are associated with each enzyme. Use the categorical chart of blood chemistry analytes (see Table 6-3 in the textbook) at the end of the chapter to locate the diseases.

Enzyme Abbreviation	Enzyme	Affected Organs and Associated Diseases
1.		
2.		
3.		
4.		
5.		
6.		

64. List the four electrolyte abbreviations found at the beginning of the chapter and state whether they are cations or anions. (Hint: They have positive or negative charges after their abbreviations.)

Electrolyte Abbreviation	Electrolyte	Cation/Anion (+/−)
1.		
2.		
3.		
4.		

115

Chapter **6** **Chemistry**

Copyright © 2015, 2011, 2006 by Saunders, an imprint of Elsevier, Inc. All rights reserved.

Procedure 6-1: Glucometer Procedure

Person evaluated _____   Date _____

Evaluated by _____   Score _____

Outcome goal	To perform FDA-approved CLIA-waived glucose test following the most current OSHA safety guidelines and applying correct quality control
Conditions	Supplies needed: - CONTOUR monitor (previously Ascensia Elite) or One Touch Test Strips - Coded test strip and liquid control - Lancet, alcohol, gauze, bandage - Personal protective equipment
Standards	Required time: 5 minutes Performance time: _____ Total possible points = _____ Points earned = _____

Evaluation Rubric Codes:
S = Satisfactory, meets standard   **U** = Unsatisfactory, fails to meet standard

NOTE: Steps marked with an asterisk (*) are critical to achieve required competency.

Preparation	Scores	
	S	**U**
A. Test information		
- Kit or instrument method: **Contour or OneTouch Ultra**		
- Manufacturer: **Bayer or LifeScan**		
- Proper storage (e.g., temperature, light): **test strips and controls are stored at room temperature**		
- Expiration date _____		
- Lot #: _____ Calibration #: _____		
- Package insert or test flow chart available: _____ yes _____ no		
B. Personal protective equipment: **gloves, gown, biohazard container**		
C. Specimen information		
- Type of specimen: **fasting, 2-hour postprandial, or random specimen**		
- Specimen source: **capillary blood or lavender-topped vacuum tube** (Note: gray-topped tubes are not used for this method.)		
- Specimen testing device: **coded test strips**		
D. Assembled all the above, sanitized hands, and applied personal protective equipment.		

Procedure: Analytical Phase	Scores	
	S	U
E. Performed/observed quantitative quality control		
- Calibration check is done automatically when each strip is inserted.		
- (*Note:* Older versions need to set the code number on the meter based on the test strip number.)		
- Control levels: Normal _____ High _____		
- (Manufacturer recommendation: Run normal control with each new batch of strips, with each new operator, and then weekly.)		
F. Performed patient test		
1. Turned on meter by inserting test strip's end with the contact bars.		
2. Stuck finger and *touched the end of the strip into the drop* of blood, allowing the blood to flow ("sip") into the strip without interruption.		
- Did **not** smear or place blood on top or bottom of strip.		
3. When beep was heard, removed the glucometer and strip away from drop of blood.		
4. Result displayed on the screen.		
*Accurate Results _____ Instructor Confirmation _____		

Follow-up: Postanalytical Phase	Scores	
	S	U
*G. Proper documentation		
1. On control log: _____ yes _____ no		
2. On patient log: _____ yes _____ no		
3. Documentation on patient chart (see following page)		
H. Identified "critical values" and took appropriate steps to notify physician		
- Expected ranges for glucose based on ADA recommendations		

	Fasting	2-Hour	Postprandial (After Drinking a Glucose-Rich Beverage)
Normal		Less than 100 mg/dL	140 mg/dL
Prediabetes		T body:100-125 mg/dL	140-199 mg/dL
Diabetes		$\geq$126 mg/dL	$\geq$200 mg/dL

	Scores	
I. Proper disposal and disinfection		
1. Disposed of all sharps in biohazard sharps containers.		
2. Disposed of all other regulated medical waste in biohazard bags.		
3. Disinfected test area and instruments according to OSHA guidelines.		
4. Sanitized hands after removing gloves.		
Total Points per Column		

Patient Name: _____

Patient Chart Entry: (Include when, what, how, why, any additional information, and the signature of the person charting.)

_____

_____

_____

Procedure 6-2: A₁c NOW+ Glycosylated Hemoglobin Procedure

Person evaluated _____ Date _____

Evaluated by _____ Score _____

Outcome goal	To perform FDA-approved glycosylated hemoglobin A_{1c} waived test following the most current OSHA safety guidelines and applying the correct quality control
Conditions	Supplies needed: - Gauze, bandage, alcohol swab - Lancet for capillary blood sample or heparin tube with venous blood sample - Sample dilution kit containing capillary tube collector and sampler body - Test cartridge - A_{1c} monitor programmed to work only with the 20 cartridges in the kit - Personal protective equipment
Standards	Required time: 5 minutes Performance time: _____ Total possible points = _____ Points earned = _____

Evaluation Rubric Codes:
S = Satisfactory, meets standard   **U** = Unsatisfactory, fails to meet standard

NOTE: Steps marked with an asterisk (*) are critical to achieve required competency.

Preparation: Preanalytical Phase	Scores S	Scores U
A. Test information		
- Kit or instrument method: **A₁cNOW+ test kit method**		
- Manufacturer: **Bayer**		
- Proper storage (e.g., temperature, light): **Foil-wrapped cartridges and kits are refrigerated. Allow 1 hour to warm to room temperature.**		
- Expiration date: _____		
- Lot # of cartridges: _____		
- Package insert or test flow chart available: _____ yes _____ no		
B. Personal protective equipment: **gloves, gown, face shield**		
C. Proper specimen used for test		
- Use only **fresh capillary blood** or venous whole blood collected in a **green heparin tube**. Venous blood can be used only if the tube is less than 1 week old and has been refrigerated during that time. Ensure blood in heparin tube is well mixed and at room temperature.		
- Specimen testing device: microcapillary tube provided in kit. After the glass capillary tube has been filled with the specimen, the analysis must begin within 5 minutes.		
D. Assembled all the above and ensured they were at the same temperature (within 18° C to 28° C), sanitized hands, and applied personal protective equipment		

Procedure: Analytical Phase	Scores	
	S	U
E. Performed/observed quantitative quality control		
- Optics check: Each box of test kits has already set its optics (make sure code on cartridge matches the code on monitor, but do not open until just before inserting into monitor).		
- Control levels: normal _____ abnormal _____		
F. Performed patient test		
1. Removed the blood collector from the foil #1 sampler dilution kit and gently touched the tip of the capillary tube that was attached to the holder into the small drop of blood from the finger stick or the venous blood drop on the slide.		
- The blood should fill the small glass capillary tube without touching the plastic holder.		
2. Wiped the sides of the capillary tube with tissue.		
3. Fully inserted the capillary holder into the sampler body that also came from the #1 sampler dilution kit (pushed together and twisted until the holder and sampler body snapped into place).		
4. Mixed sample with the dilution by tilting 6 to 8 times; stood the sampler on the table.		
5. Opened the #2 test cartridge foil package and performed the following within 2 minutes:		
- Clicked the cartridge into the monitor that came in the same kit box; checked code numbers, which must match.		
- While the monitor indicated "WAIT," prepared the sample by removing the base.		
- Did not add the sample until the monitor indicated "SMPL."		
- Pushed sampler down onto the white well of the cartridge.		
- The monitor was on a level surface and was not moved until the test was complete.		
6. After several minutes, the monitor indicated "QCOK," followed by the test result and by the number of tests left in the kit.		
7. Recorded the results from the display and reported to the physician.		
*Accurate Results _____ Instructor Confirmation _____		

Follow-up: Postanalytical Phase	Scores	
	S	U
*G. Proper documentation		
1. Control logs: _____ yes _____ no		
2. Patient log: _____ yes _____ no		
3. Documentation on patient chart (see following page).		
4. Identified critical values and took appropriate steps to notify physician.		
- Expected values:		

Nondiabetics	3%-6%
Controlled diabetics	6%-8%
Poorly controlled diabetics	20% or higher
Note: Because A_{1c} is also affected by the hemoglobin concentration, normal ranges should be determined by each laboratory to conform to the population being tested.	

H. Proper disposal and disinfection		
1. Disposed of the cartridge in biohazard sharps containers, and returned monitor to the box for subsequent testing.		
2. Disposed of all other regulated medical waste in biohazard bags.		
3. Disinfected test area and instruments according to OSHA guidelines.		
4. Sanitized hands after removing gloves.		
Total Points per Column		

6-2

Patient Name: _____

Patient Chart Entry: (Include when, what, how, why, any additional information, and the signature of the person charting.)

_____

_____

_____

Procedure 6-3: Cholestech Method of Measuring Lipids and Glucose

Person evaluated _____ Date _____

Evaluated by _____ Score _____

Outcome goal	To perform FDA-approved lipid profile waived test following the most current OSHA safety guidelines and applying the correct quality control.
Conditions	Supplies needed: - Optics check cassette - Level 1 and 2 liquid controls - Alcohol, gauze, and lancets or vacuum lithium heparin tubes - Capillary tubes and plungers for finger stick sample - Mini-Pet pipette and pipette tips for venipuncture sample - Personal protective equipment
Standards	Required time: 10 minutes Performance time: _____ Total possible points = _____ Points earned = _____

Evaluation Rubric Codes:
S = Satisfactory, meets standard   **U** = Unsatisfactory, fails to meet standard

NOTE: Steps marked with an asterisk (*) are critical to achieve required competency.

Preparation: Preanalytical Phase	Scores	
	S	U
A. Test information		
- Kit or instrument method: **Cholestech LDX Analyzer**		
- Manufacturer: **Cholestech Corporation**		
- Proper storage (e.g., temperature, light): **Foil-wrapped cassettes are refrigerated. They must return to room temperature before testing.**		
- Expiration date: _____		
- Cassette lot #: _____		
- Package insert or test flow chart available: _____ yes _____ no		
B. Personal protective equipment: **gloves, gown, biohazard containers**		
C. Specimen information		
- Patient preparation: **Fasting recommended for cholesterol. Triglyceride requires fasting and no alcohol consumption in previous 48 hours.**		
- Type of specimen: **capillary blood or lithium heparin (green) tube only for venous blood**		
- Specimen testing device: **Cholestech capillary tube (once in tube, must be tested within 5 minutes)**		
D. Assembled all the above, sanitized hands, and applied personal protective equipment		

Procedure: Analytical Phase	Scores	
	S	U
E. Performed/observed quantitative quality control		
- Calibration check: **Run calibration cassette daily.**		
- Control levels: **Level 1, Level 2** (Use the mini-Pet pipettes provided by Cholestech)		

F. Performed patient test		
1. Allowed cassette to come to room temperature (at least 10 minutes before opening).		
2. Made sure analyzer was plugged in and warmed up.		
3. Removed cassette from its pouch and placed it on flat surface.		
- Held cassette by the short sides only.		
- Did not touch the black bar or the brown magnetic strip.		
4. Pressed RUN; the analyzer did a self-test, and the screen displayed "selftest running" and then "selftest OK."		
5. The cassette drawer opened, and the screen displayed "load cassette and press RUN."		
- Drawer remains open for 4 minutes, after which it closes with the message "System time-out: RUN to continue." If the RUN button is not pushed within 15 seconds, the drawer closes, and the screen goes blank. Press RUN again, allow to go through the self-test again, and proceed.		
6. Collected fresh capillary blood to the black line of the capillary tube with plunger inserted into the red end of the tube.		
- Or collected fresh venous whole blood with the Cholestech mini-Pet pipette.		
7. Placed whole blood sample into the test cassette sample well.		
- The finger stick sample must be put into the cassette within 5 minutes of collection or the blood will clot.		
8. *Immediately* placed cassette into the drawer of the analyzer.		
- Kept cassette level after the sample was applied.		
- The black reaction bar faced toward the analyzer.		
- The brown magnetic strip was on the right.		
9. Pressed RUN. The drawer closed, and the screen displayed "[test names]—running."		
10. When the test was completed, the analyzer beeped, and the screen displayed results at the same time the printer printed results. (Press DATA to display the calculated results of all tests on the screen if running a panel of tests.)		

*Accurate Results _____ Instructor Confirmation _____

Follow-up: Postanalytical Phase	Scores	
	S	U
*G. Proper documentation _____		
1. On control log: _____ yes _____ no		
2. On patient log: _____ yes _____ no		
3. Documented on patient chart (see below).		
4. Identified "critical values" and took appropriate steps to notify physician.		

NCEP ATP III guidelines for lipid panels:

Test	Desirable
Total cholesterol (TC)	<200 mg/dL
HDL cholesterol	>40 mg/dL
LDL cholesterol	<130 mg/dL
Triglycerides	<150 mg/dL
TC/HDL ratio	≤4.5
Glucose	Fasting: 60-110 mg/dL
	Nonfasting: <160 mg/dL
Alanine aminotransferase	10-40 U/L

H. Proper disposal and disinfection		
1. Disposed of all sharps into biohazard sharps containers.		
2. Disposed of all other regulated medical waste into biohazard bags.		
3. Disinfected test area and instruments according to OSHA guidelines.		
4. Sanitized hands after removing gloves.		
Total Points per Column		

Patient Name: _____

Attach printed readout, or record results on the chart provided:

Test	Results	Desirable
Total cholesterol (TC)		<200 mg/dL
HDL cholesterol		>40 mg/dL
LDL cholesterol		<130 mg/dL
Triglycerides		<150 mg/dL
TC/HDL ratio		≤4.5
Other		
Glucose		Fasting: 60-110 mg/dL
		Nonfasting: <160 mg/dL

Procedure 6-4: i-STAT Chemistry Analyzer Procedure

Person evaluated _____ Date _____

Evaluated by _____ Score _____

Outcome goal	To perform FDA-approved i-STAT chemistry waived test following the most current OSHA safety guidelines and applying the correct quality control
Conditions	Supplies needed: - i-STAT 1 handheld, recharging dock, and printer - Ampule of Level 1 liquid control for i-STAT CHEM 8+ - i-STAT CHEM 8+ cartridges - Fresh blood collected in lithium heparin tubes (green top) - 1-mL plain syringe - Safety transfer device or safety tip - Personal protective equipment and biohazard container
Standards	Required time: 15 minutes Performance time: _____ Total possible points = _____ Points earned = _____

Evaluation Rubric Codes:
S = Satisfactory, meets standard   **U** = Unsatisfactory, fails to meet standard

NOTE: Steps marked with an asterisk (*) are critical to achieve required competency.

Preparation: Preanalytical Phase	Scores	
	S	**U**
A. Test information		
- Kit or instrument method: **i-STAT Chemistry Analyzer**		
- Manufacturer: **Abbott**		
- Proper storage (e.g., temperature, light): **Foil-wrapped cartridges and controls are refrigerated. They must return to room temperature before testing.**		
- Expiration date: _____		
- Scan cartridge lot #: _____		
- Package insert or test flow chart available: _____ yes _____ no		
B. Personal protective equipment: **gloves, gown, biohazard containers**		
C. Specimen information		
- Patient preparation: **Collect blood, ensuring the 4-mL heparin tube fills completely and is mixed by tilting 10 times. Specimen should be tested within 10 minutes.**		
- Type of specimen: **Lithium heparin (green) tube only for venous blood**		
- Specimen testing device: **A 1-mL syringe is used to remove the specimen from the green vacuum tube and transfer the blood to the cartridge.**		
D. Assembled all the above, sanitized hands, and applied personal protective equipment.		

Procedure: Analytical Phase	Scores	
	S	U
E. Performed/observed quantitative quality control		
- Calibration check: **Use the simulator provided by i-STAT.**		
- Control level: **Level 1 ampule is provided by i-STAT.**		
F. Performed patient test		
1. Allowed cassette to come to room temperature (at least 10 minutes before opening).		
2. Keyed in operator and patient information into the handheld analyzer, followed by scanning the cartridge bar code until a beep was heard.		
3. *Within 10 minutes* of drawing a 4-mL specimen of blood into a vacuum tube, performed the following:		
- Mixed the specimen by tilting 10 times.		
- Connected a safety tip or safety transfer device to a 1-mL syringe.		
- Inverted the green-top tube with the specimen and pierced the green stopper with the syringe safety tip or the transfer device.		
- *Slowly* pulled back on the syringe plunger until it was about one half full; noted any air bubbles that entered syringe while transferring and did not push them back into specimen.		
- Disconnected syringe from vacuum tube and continued to hold it with tip pointed upward; held a gauze pad at tip to absorb blood while syringe plunger slowly pushed out the air and approximately 3 drops of blood.		
- Tore open the foiled cartridge pouch and removed the cartridge by holding the sides and placed it on a flat surface.		
- Held the syringe tip directly over sample well and carefully pushed the blood into the cartridge until the blood reached the arrow, and there was still blood remaining in the well but not overflowing.		
4. Moved the tab over the well from left to right using one finger; did not press on the beige circle area directly over the well; pushed down on the tab until it snapped into place.		
5. Used the grooved area to the left of the well or the sides of the cartridge to insert it slowly into the analyzer.		
- The handheld first displayed "Identifying Cartridge" and then a time-to-result bar.		
- ***Did not*** **remove cartridge until the "Cartridge Locked" message was removed and results were displayed on screen.**		
6. Reviewed results		
- After 2 to 3 minutes, the results appeared on the screen. The "→ Page" command on bottom of the screen indicated more results would appear on a second screen. Pressed the print button to send the results to the printer by wireless transmission or by the docking device USB connection.		
- The handheld showed the numerical values and units with the results. It also showed bar graphs with tic marks for reference ranges.		
*Accurate Results _____ Instructor Confirmation _____		

Follow-up: Postanalytical Phase	Scores	
	S	**U**
*G. Proper documentation		
1. On control log: _____ yes _____ no		
2. On patient log: _____ yes _____ no		
3. Documented on patient chart (see below).		
4. Identified "critical values" and took appropriate steps to notify physician.		
*See table of test ranges below.		
H. Proper disposal and disinfection		
1. Disposed of all sharps in biohazard sharps containers.		
2. Disposed of all other regulated medical waste in biohazard bags.		
3. Disinfected test area and instruments according to OSHA guidelines.		
4. Sanitized hands after removing gloves.		
Total Points per Column		

Test	Test Symbol	Units	Reportable Range	Reference Range	Results	Critical Low/High
Sodium	Na	mmol/L	100-180	138-146		
Potassium	K	mmol/L	2.0-9.0	3.5-4.9		
Chloride	Cl	mmol/L	65-140	98-109		
Total carbon dioxide	TCO_2	mmol/L	5-50	24-29		
Ionized calcium	iCa	mmol/L	0.25-2.50	1.12-1.32		
Glucose	Glu	mg/dL	20-700	70-105		
Urea nitrogen	BUN	mg/dL	3-140	8-26		
Creatinine	Crea	mg/dL	0.2-20.0	0.6-1.3		
Hematocrit	Hct	% PCV	10-75	38-51		
Hemoglobin*	Hb	g/dL	3.4-25.5	12-17		
Anion gap*	AnGap	mmol/L	10-99	10-20		

Patient Name: _____

Attach printed readout, or record results on the chart above.

129

Procedure 6-7: Occult Blood: iFOB Method

Person evaluated _____   Date _____

Evaluated by _____   Score _____

Outcome goal	To perform FDA-approved, CLIA-waived fecal occult blood test using the most current OSHA safety guidelines and applying the correct quality control
Conditions	Supplies needed: **Patient supplies for collecting fecal specimen at home:** a. step-by-step illustrated instruction sheet; b. specimen collection paper to place across toilet seat; c. specimen collection tube with internal sampling probe to pierce the specimen; d. plastic biohazard bag and mailer to send specimen to the laboratory or office. **In-office testing cassette:** foil-wrapped testing cassette

Evaluation Rubric Codes:
S = Satisfactory, meets standard   **U** = Unsatisfactory, fails to meet standard

NOTE: Steps marked with an asterisk (*) are critical to achieve required competency.

A. Preparation: Preanalytical Phase	Scores	
	S	U
1. Test information		
- Kit or instrument method: **iFOB**		
- Manufacturer: **QuickVue by Quidel**		
- Proper storage (e.g., temperature, light): **room temperature**		
- Expiration date: _____		
- Lot # on kit: _____		
- Package insert or test flow chart available: _____ yes _____ no		
2. Instructed patient on the following dietary preparations:		
The QuickVue iFOB test is specific to human hemoglobin, and the patient does not need to follow the food restrictions of other fecal occult test methods. However, patients with the following conditions should not be considered for testing because these conditions may interfere with test results:		
- Menstrual bleeding		
- Bleeding hemorrhoids		
- Constipation bleeding		
- Urinary bleeding		
Patients with the above conditions may be considered for testing after bleeding ceases.		
- Alcohol and certain medications such as aspirin, indomethacin, reserpine, phenylbutazone, corticosteroids, and nonsteroidal anti-inflammatory drugs may also cause gastrointestinal irritation and subsequent bleeding in some patients.		
3. Enter the patient identification information on the collection tube label.		

1 5

4. At home collection performed by patient:		
a. When collecting specimens, the patient should follow the take-home instructions as follows:		
- Do not collect specimen if bleeding is present from hemorrhoids, constipation, urination, or menstruation.		
- Urinate before positioning collection paper (or a paper plate)		
- Do not urinate on fecal specimen or collection paper		
- Position paper on rear half of toilet seat and press the tape down on each side		
- Deposit fecal specimen on the collection paper		
b. Unscrew the dark blue Sampler probe from the collection tube that contains a liquid buffer solution.		
- Using the probe, pierce the specimen in at least five different sites.		
- Insert the sampler back into the collection tube, firmly tighten, and shake the tube well.		
- Flush remaining specimen and collection paper		
c. Make sure patient ID line on the tube has the proper name on the label. Then insert the collection tube that has the well-mixed specimen and solution into:		
- absorbent sleeve,		
- then plastic specimen pouch,		
- then into the cardboard mailer.		
- Mail or bring the specimen to the medical office or laboratory.		

	Scores	
B. Procedure: Analytical Phase Performed in the Office	**S**	**U**
Test performed in office.		
1. Apply gloves, and observe Universal Precautions. Confirm that all necessary information was written on the collection tube.		
2. Shake tube well and unscrew pale blue cap		
3. Cover the exposed tip with the absorbent sleeve or gauze, and snap the tip away.		
4. Squeeze 6 drops into the test well.		
5. Read results as positive or negative or invalid after 5 to 10 minutes based on the following criteria:		
- Positive result: A pink line appears next to the letter "T" and next to the letter "C."		
- Negative result: Only one pink line forms next to the letter "C."		
6. Invalid test: If there is no pink line next to the letter "C," the test results are invalid and should not be reported.		
*Accurate Results _____ Instructor Confirmation _____		

C. Follow-up: Postanalytical Phase	Scores	
	S	U
Proper documentation		
1. On control/patient log: _____ yes _____ no		
2. Documented on patient chart (see following page).		
3. Identified critical values and took appropriate steps to notify physician.		
- Expected values for occult blood: negative		
Proper disposal and disinfection		
1. Disposed of all regulated medical waste in biohazard bags		
2. Disinfected test area and instruments according to OSHA guidelines.		
3. Sanitized hands after removing gloves.		
Total Points per Column		

6-7

Patient Name: _____

Patient Chart Entry: (Include when, what, how, why, any additional information, and the signature of the person charting.)

_____

_____

_____

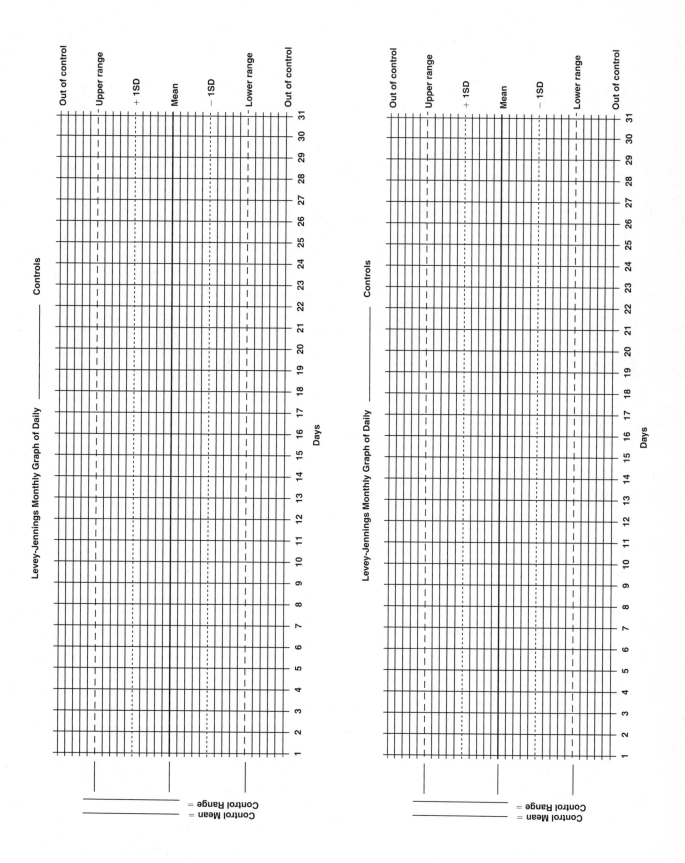

7 Immunology

VOCABULARY REVIEW

Match each definition with the correct term.

_____ 1. B-lymphocytic cell response to antigens resulting in the production of specific antibodies to destroy a foreign invader; also called antibody-mediated immunity

_____ 2. Cells capable of engulfing and ingesting microorganisms and cellular debris

_____ 3. Compound released by injured cells that causes dilation of blood vessels

_____ 4. Immunoglobulins produced specifically to destroy foreign invaders

_____ 5. Long-term protection against future infections resulting from the production of antibodies formed naturally during an infection or artificially by vaccination

_____ 6. Nonpathogenic microorganisms that normally inhabit the skin and mucous membranes

_____ 7. Overall reaction of the body to tissue injury or invasion by an infectious agent; characterized by redness, heat, swelling, and pain

_____ 8. Process of engulfing and digesting microorganisms and cellular debris

_____ 9. Proteins secreted by infected cells to prevent further replication and spread of an infection into neighboring cells

_____ 10. Proteins that stimulate phagocytosis and inflammation and are capable of destroying bacteria

_____ 11. Short-term acquired immunity created by antibodies received naturally through the placenta (or the colostrum to an infant) or artificially by injection

_____ 12. Special type of lymphocyte that attacks and destroys infected cells and cancer cells in a nonspecific way

_____ 13. Substances that are perceived as foreign to the body and elicit an antibody response

_____ 14. T-lymphocytic cell response to antigens

_____ 15. Thin sheets of tissue that line the internal cavities and canals of the body and serve as a barrier against the entry of pathogens

_____ 16. Destructive tissue diseases caused by antibody/self-antigen reactions

A. active immunity
B. autoimmune diseases
C. antibodies
D. antigens
E. cell-mediated immunity
F. complement proteins
G. histamine
H. humoral immunity
I. inflammation
J. interferons
K. mucous membrane
L. natural killer cells
M. normal flora
N. passive immunity
O. phagocytes
P. phagocytosis

Match the B and T lymphocytes with their functions.

_____ 17. Antigen-activated B lymphocytes that remember an identified antigen for future encounters

_____ 18. Antigen-activated lymphocytes that attack foreign antigens directly and destroy cells that bear the antigens; also called cytotoxic cells

_____ 19. Antigen-activated lymphocytes that inhibit T and B cells after enough cells have been activated

_____ 20. Antigen-activated lymphocytes that stimulate other T cells and help B cells produce antibodies

_____ 21. Antigen-activated T lymphocytes that remember an antigen for future encounters

_____ 22. Subgroup of B lymphocytes that produce the antibodies that travel through the blood specifically targeting and reacting with antigens

A. killer T cells
B. suppressor T cells
C. plasma cells
D. helper T cells (T_H4 or CD4)
E. memory B cells
F. memory T cells

Match the immunology testing and disease terms with the correct definition.

_____ 23. Antibody that appears during an Epstein-Barr viral infection (mononucleosis) that has an unusual affinity to heterophile antigens on sheep red cells

_____ 24. Branch of laboratory medicine that performs antibody/antigen testing with serum

_____ 25. Clumping together of blood cells or latex beads caused by antibodies adhering to their antigens

_____ 26. A hemolytic anemia in newborns resulting from maternal-fetal blood group incompatibility

_____ 27. Testing in a laboratory apparatus

_____ 28. Pertaining to a visual color change that appears when an enzyme-linked antibody/antigen reaction occurs

_____ 29. Pertaining to the attachment of an antigen or antibody to a solid surface such as latex beads, wells in plastic dishes, or plastic cartridges

_____ 30. Process of injecting harmless or killed microorganisms into the body to induce immunity against a potential pathogen; also called immunization

_____ 31. Raised induration

_____ 32. Substances within the body that induce the production of antibodies that attack an individual's own body tissues; also called autoantigens

_____ 33. A quantitative test that measures the amount of antibody that reacts with a specific antigen

_____ 34. Testing within a host or living organism

A. agglutination
B. chromatographic
C. erythroblastosis fetalis
D. heterophile antibody
E. immunosorbent
F. in vitro
G. in vivo
H. self-antigens
I. serology
J. titer
K. vaccination
L. wheal

142

Chapter **7** **Immunology**

Copyright © 2015, 2011, 2006 by Saunders, an imprint of Elsevier, Inc. All rights reserved.

35. When a pathogen is invading the body, list two examples of protection for each line of defense:

    First line of external defenses: _____

    Second line of internal, nonspecific defenses: _____

    _____

    Third line of internal, specific defenses: _____

    _____

36. List two white cells that are phagocytic.

    _____

37. Give an example of a normal flora organism, and describe how it prevents the invasion of pathogens.

    _____

    _____

38. List the clinical signs of inflammation.

    _____

39. Describe antigens.

    _____

    _____

40. Which cells are associated with cell-mediated immunity?

    _____

41. What is another name for antibodies? (Hint: They are a subcategory of proteins.)

    _____

42. Name the five types of antibodies by their immunoglobulin identification.

    _____

43. Refer to Figure 7-4A and B in the textbook and give examples of natural and artificial active immunity and natural and artificial passive immunity.

    _____

    _____

44. The pregnancy test determines the presence of what antigenic substance?

_____

_____

45. Fill in the blanks for the following medical information regarding infectious mononucleosis:

Causative agent: _____

Clinical symptoms: _____

Hematology findings: _____

Immunology findings: _____

46. Label the QuickVue+ infectious mononucleosis supplies (see Procedure 7-2 in the textbook).

47. Describe the relationship between *Helicobacter pylori* and ulcers.

_____

_____

48. Indicate whether the following statements about HIV are TRUE or FALSE.

_____ a. HIV is now a curable disease.

_____ b. ARV (antiretroviral) is a medication that destroys HIV.

_____ c. Self-testing for HIV is now available.

_____ d. It is possible to receive a false-positive or a false-negative HIV test result.

49. Label the HIV supplies needed to perform the Uni-Gold Recombigen HIV blood test (see Procedure 7-4 in the textbook).

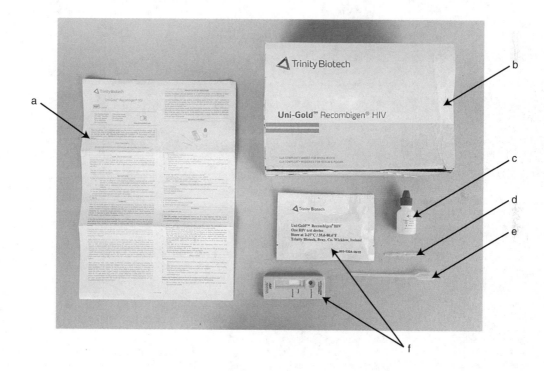

50. Based on the test results illustrated in the following chart, interpret the results for each test as **positive, negative,** or **invalid** based on the interpretation directions found in the textbook referenced figures.

	Test	Figure in Textbook	Interpreted Result
A		ICON hCG Figure 7-6	
B		hCG Procedure 7-1, *B*	
C		Infectious Mononucleosis Procedure 7-2, *D*	

	Test	Figure in Textbook	Interpreted Result
D		**HIV Blood Test Procedure 7-4 Fig. H - Last Figure on the right**	
E		**HIV Blood Test Procedure 7-4 Figure G on the right (b)**	
F		**HIV Blood Test Procedure 7-4 Figure H- first fig on the left**	
G		**HIV Blood Test Procedure 7-4 Figure G– on the left (a)**	

Chapter **7** **Immunology**

51. Define agglutination.

_____

_____

52. Define immunohematology, and give three reasons why testing is done in this area.

_____

_____

53. Give the antigens and antibodies found in type AB blood. (See Table 7-2.)

_____

54. Would a woman with D antigen on her red blood cells be considered Rh positive or Rh negative? _____

    Would she be at risk for hemolytic disease of the newborn? _____

55. When the body is exposed to the following pathogens, it produces specific antibodies that can be measured in the plasma or serum. Refer to Table 7-3 in the textbook, identify the following pathogenic diseases, and indicate whether the pathogen is a bacteria or virus.

Pathogen	Disease	Bacteria or Virus
RSV		
Rubella		
Chlamydia		
Varicella zoster		
B. burgdorferi		

56. List three cancers that can be detected by immunologic testing (see Table 7-3 in the textbook).

_____

_____

Procedure 7-2: QuickVue+ Mononucleosis Test Procedure

Person evaluated _____ Date _____

Evaluated by _____ Score/Grade _____

Outcome goal	To perform FDA-approved CLIA-waived infectious mononucleosis test following the most current OSHA safety guidelines and applying the correct quality control

Conditions	Supplies needed:
	- QuickVue test kit containing:
	- Developer
	  - Individually wrapped reaction units
	  - Capillary tubes for capillary blood and pipettes for venous blood
	  - Positive and negative liquid controls
	  - Instruction insert and pictorial flow chart
	- Other materials needed:
	  - Capillary puncture supplies (lancet, alcohol, gauze, bandage), or whole blood venipuncture specimen
	  - Timer
	  - Personal protective equipment

Standards	Required time: 10 minutes Performance time: _____ Total possible points = _____ Points earned = _____

Evaluation Rubric Codes:
S = Satisfactory, meets standard   **U** = Unsatisfactory, fails to meet standard

NOTE: Steps marked with an asterisk (*) are critical to achieve required competency.

Preparation for Mononucleosis Test: Preanalytical Phase	Scores	
	S	**U**
A. Test information		
- Kit method: **QuickVue+ Mononucleosis Test**		
- Manufacturer: **Quidel**		
- Proper storage (e.g., temperature, light): **room temperature**		
- Lot # of kit: _____		
- Expiration date: _____		
- Package insert or test flow chart available: _____ yes _____ no		
B. Personal protective equipment: gloves, gown, biohazard container		
C. Specimen information		
- Use the capillary transfer tube provided in the kit to obtain capillary blood or the larger transfer pipette in the kit to obtain the venipuncture whole blood and the liquid controls.		

151

Procedure for Mononucleosis: Analytical Phase	S	U
D. Performed/observed qualitative quality control		
- External liquid controls: positive _____ negative _____		
- Internal control: **The color blue fills the "read result" window.**		
E. Performed patient test		
1. Dispensed all the blood from the capillary tube into the "add" well or transferred a large drop from the venous whole blood specimen with the pipette.		
2. Added 5 drops of developer to the "add" well.		
- Held bottle vertical and allowed drops to fall freely.		
3. Read results at 5 minutes.		
- "Test complete" line must be visible by 10 minutes.		
4. Interpretation of results (circled result):		
- Positive = Any shade of a blue vertical line forms a positive (+) sign in the "read result" window along with the blue "test complete" line. Even a faint blue vertical line should be reported as a positive result.		
- Negative = No blue vertical line appears in the "read result" window along with the blue "test complete" line.		
- Invalid = After 10 minutes, no signal is observed in the "test complete" window, or the color blue fills the "read result" window. If either occurs, the test must be repeated with a new reaction unit. If the problem continues, contact technical support.		
*Accurate Results _____ Instructor Confirmation _____		

Follow-up: Postanalytical Phase	Scores	
	S	U
*F. Proper documentation		
1. On control/patient log: _____ yes _____ no		
2. Documented on patient chart (see below).		
3. Identified critical values and took appropriate steps to notify physician.		
- Expected values for analyte: negative for mononucleosis		
G. Proper disposal and disinfection		
1. Disposed of all sharps in biohazard sharps containers.		
2. Disposed of all other regulated medical waste in biohazard bags.		
3. Disinfected test area and instruments according to OSHA guidelines.		
4. Sanitized hands after removing gloves.		
Total Points per Column		

Patient Name: _____

Patient Chart Entry: (Include when, what, how, why, any additional information, and the signature of the person charting.)

_____

_____

_____

Procedure 7-4: Uni-Gold Recombigen HIV Blood Test

Person evaluated _____ Date _____

Evaluated by _____ Score/Grade _____

Outcome goal	To perform FDA-approved CLIA-waived **Uni-Gold Recombigen HIV Blood Test** following the most current OSHA safety guidelines and applying the correct quality control

Conditions	Supplies needed:
	- Uni-Gold test kit containing:
	  - Package insert and patient information sheets
	  - Box with 20 test devices
	  - Wash solution
	  - Finger stick sample collection and transfer pipette
	  - Disposable pipette to use with venipuncture whole blood
	  - Foil pouch and its test device
	  - Positive and negative controls
	  - Timer
	  - Personal protective equipment

Standards	Required time: 10 to 15 minutes (depending on blood collection method) Performance time: _____ Total possible points = _____ Points earned = _____

Evaluation Rubric Codes:
S = Satisfactory, meets standard **U** = Unsatisfactory, fails to meet standard

NOTE: Steps marked with an asterisk (*) are critical to achieve required competency.

Preparation for Uni-Gold Recombigen HIV Blood Test: Preanalytical Phase	Scores	
	S	**U**
A. Test information		
- Kit method: **Uni-Gold Recombigen HIV Blood Test**		
- Manufacturer: **Trinity Biotech**		
- Proper storage (e.g., temperature, light): **room temperature**		
- Lot # of kit: _____		
- Expiration date: _____		
- Package insert or test flow chart available: _____ yes _____		
B. Personal protective equipment: gloves, gown, face mask, biohazard containers		
C. Specimen information		
- Use the capillary transfer tube provided in the kit to obtain capillary blood or the larger transfer pipette in the kit to obtain the venipuncture whole blood and the liquid controls.		
Procedure for Uni-Gold Recombigen HIV Blood Test: Analytical Phase	**S**	**U**
D. Performed/observed qualitative quality control		
- External liquid controls: positive _____ negative _____		
- Internal control: **The red line next to "CONTROL"**		
E. Performed patient test		
1. Sanitized hands, and applied personal protective equipment.		
2. Documented that the information sheet has been given to the patient and that the patient has read it.		

3. Allow the unopened foil packet and wash solution to come to room temperature. PERFORM ONLY ONE TEST AT A TIME.		
4. Open kit and lay the testing device on a clean flat surface.		
5. Label the device with the appropriate patient information.		
6. Collect the sample via venipuncture using EDTA (lavender tube) or heparin (green tube). Or, alternatively, collect the sample from a finger stick using the appropriate provided transfer pipette until the blood reaches the mark. It is important to hold the pipette gently in a horizontal position and allow the blood to fill to the mark on the pipette.		
7. Add 1 free flowing drop of the venous whole blood to the sample port (using the proper disposable transfer pipette in the kit). Or, alternatively, immediately dispense all the blood in the capillary pipette from the finger stick into the sample port. Note: Both of the above procedures should be done with a barrier shield or a full face mask to protect the operator from possible blood exposure to the mucous membranes.		
8. Discard the pipette in biohazard waste.		
9. Hold the dropper bottle of wash solution above the sample port in a vertical position, and add 4 free flowing drops of the wash solution to the sample port.		
10. Do not move the test cassette until the assay is complete. Read and record the results of the test after 10 minutes but not more than 12 minutes: a. **Negative result**: Only one red line forms next to "Control." b. **Positive result**: A pink/red line appears next to "Test" and next to "Control." Report as "Preliminary Positive." c. **Invalid results**: For a test to be valid, a pink/red control line must be present, and the sample port must show a full red color. Refer to Fig. H in the Text Procedure 7-4 for the five possible invalid results. If any of these results appear, do not report the patient result. The test must be repeated with a new testing device.		
*Accurate Results _____ Instructor Confirmation _____		

Follow-up: Postanalytical Phase	Scores	
	S	**U**
11. Discard all the test materials in the appropriate biohazard containers.		
12. Remove and discard gloves in the biohazard container, and sanitize the hands.		
13. Proper documentation		
■ On control/patient log: _____ yes _____ no		
■ Documented on patient chart (see below).		
■ Identified critical values and took appropriate steps to notify physician.		
- Expected values for analyte: negative		
Total Points per Column		

Patient Name: _____

Patient Chart Entry: (Include when, what, how, why, any additional information, and the signature of the person charting.)

_____

_____

_____

Procedure 7-5: HIV OraQuick Test

Person evaluated _____ Date _____

Evaluated by _____ Score/Grade _____

Outcome goal	To perform FDA-approved CLIA-waived HIV OraQuick Test following the most current OSHA safety guidelines and applying the correct quality control

Conditions	**OraQuick HIV self-test kit contents:**
	- Box and its white plastic test kit containing the flip chart directions and the following displayed items located in the pull out drawer:
	   - Required manufacturer's insert and pencil for writing start and finish times
	   - Plastic bag for disposal of the test supplies when finished
	   - Foil-wrapped test stick and test tube
	   - Two booklets titled "Please Read this Book First—HIV, Testing, and Me" and "What Your Results Mean to You!"
	Additional items (if performing the HIV OraQuick Test in the office):
	- Positive and negative external liquid controls
	- Personal protective equipment including gloves, face protection, gown, and OSHA disposal equipment

Standards	Required time: minutes 30 to 50 minutes (based on setting up test and incubation time of 20 to 40 minutes) Performance time: _____ Total possible points = _____ Points earned = _____

Evaluation Rubric Codes:
S = Satisfactory, meets standard   **U** = Unsatisfactory, fails to meet standard

NOTE: Steps marked with an asterisk (*) are critical to achieve required competency.

Preparation for HIV OraQuick Test: Preanalytical Phase	Scores	
	S	**U**
A. Test information		
- Kit method: **HIV OraQuick Test**		
- Manufacturer: **OraQuick**		
- Proper storage (e.g., temperature, light): **room temperature**		
- Lot # of kit: _____		
- Expiration date: _____		
- Package insert or test flow chart available: _____ yes _____ no		
B. Personal protective equipment: gloves, gown, face mask, biohazard containers		
C. Patient preparation		
- Most people feel a little bit anxious when taking an HIV test. If patients feel very anxious about taking the self-test, they may want to wait until they are calmer or get tested by a physician at a local clinic.		
- It is important not to eat, drink, or use oral care products (e.g., mouthwash, toothpaste, or whitening strips) 30 minutes before starting the test.		
- Remove dental products such as dentures or any other products that cover the gums.		
- Find a quiet, well-lit place where you can stay for at least 20 minutes.		
- You must follow the test directions carefully to get an accurate result.		
- Make sure you have a timer, watch, or something that can time 20 to 40 minutes.		

Chapter **7** Immunology

Procedure for HIV OraQuick Self-Test or In-Office Test: Analytical Phase	S	U
D. Performing the test.		
1. Sanitize the hands, and apply personal protective equipment.		
2. Ensure that the pretest booklet, "Read This First," has been given to the patient and that the patient has read it.		
3. Open kit drawer and lay out all supplies.		
4. With the white plastic lid in the open position, proceed by following the directions and demonstrations on each of the numbered flip charts:		
Step 1: Open Test Tube—Find the packet labeled "Test Tube," and tear open the packet to remove the test tube.		
Step 2: Set Up—Be careful! There's liquid at the bottom of the tube. Hold the tube upright. Gently *pop* off the test tube's cap—do not twist. Put the test tube in the holder labeled "Test Tube Holder" located on the right side of the plastic lid that is opened and upright.		
Step 3: Open Test Stick—Locate the packet labeled "Test Stick." Tear open the packet and remove the test stick being careful not to touch the pad with your fingers.		
Step 4: Swipe Gums—(Make sure the timer is ready and set for 20 minutes, but do not start it yet.) Gently swipe the pad along the upper gums once and then the lower gums once. Make sure you swipe the pad between the gum and the lips from one side all the way to the other on both the upper and the lower gums.		
Step 5: Drop in and Start Timing—Put the test stick pad directly into the test tube located on the right side of the plastic lid and start the timer for 20 minutes. Note: The kit also provides a pencil and a place to write in the start time, the time after 20 minutes, and the time after 40 minutes.		
Step 6: Wait 20 minutes—The test kit provides a flap to cover the test area on the stick. The area will turn pink for a few minutes. That is normal. Do not read the results before 20 minutes (this may give a wrong result). Read the results between 20 and 40 minutes. After 40 minutes, the test will no longer be accurate. While waiting for the results, the patient should read the second booklet, "HIV, Testing, and Me"		
Step 7: Reading Your Results—Move the flap that covered the test area to see the results. Compare the test stick with the pictures on the flip chart. If the results do not look like the examples on the flip chart or there are no lines on the test stick, the test is not working. For questions, call toll-free 1-866-436-6527. **NOTE:** A positive result with this test does not mean the person tested is definitely infected with HIV, but rather that additional testing should be done in a medical setting. A negative result with this test does not mean that a person is definitely not infected with HIV, particularly when exposure may have been within the previous 3 months.		
Step 8: Dispose—Remove the test stick, put the cap on the test tube, and place all the contents in the disposal bag provided in the test kit and throw it away. **For questions, call toll-free 1-866-436-6527**		
*Accurate Results _____ Instructor Confirmation _____		

7-5

Follow-up: Postanalytical Phase	Scores	
	S	**U**
E. Proper documentation		
■ On control/patient log: _____ yes _____ no		
■ Documented on patient chart.		
■ Identified critical values and took appropriate steps to notify physician.		
- Expected values for analyte: negative		
Total Points per Column		

Patient Name: _____

Patient Chart Entry: (Include when, what, how, why, any additional information, and the signature of the person charting.)

_____

_____

_____

GENERIC ANALYTICAL TEST FORM (FOR KITS NOT COVERED IN THE TEXTBOOK OR WORKBOOK)

Qualitative Test: _____

Person evaluated _____   Date _____

Evaluated by _____   Score/Grade _____

Outcome goal	
Conditions	Supplies required:
Standards	Required time: _____
	Performance time: _____
	Total possible points = _____ Points earned = _____
Evaluation Rubric Codes: **S** = Satisfactory, meets standard **U** = Unsatisfactory, fails to meet standard	
NOTE: Steps marked with an asterisk (*) are critical to achieve required competency.	

Preparation: Preanalytical Phase	Scores S	Scores U
A. Test information		
- Kit method:		
- Manufacturer:		
- Proper storage (e.g., temperature, light):		
- Lot # of kit: _____		
- Expiration date: _____		
- Package insert or test flow chart available: _____ yes _____ no		
B. Personal protective equipment:		
C. Specimen information		
Procedure: Analytical Phase	Scores S	Scores U
D. Performed/observed qualitative quality control		
- External liquid controls: positive _____ negative _____		
- Internal control		
E. Performed patient test		
1.		
2.		
3.		
4.		
Positive =		
Negative =		
Invalid =		
*Accurate Results _____ Instructor Confirmation _____		

Follow-up: Postanalytical Phase	Scores	
	S	U
*F. Proper documentation		
1. On control/patient log: _____ yes _____ no		
2. Documented on patient chart (see below).		
3. Identified critical values and took appropriate steps to notify physician.		
- Expected values for analyte:		
G. Proper disposal and disinfection		
1. Disposed of all sharps in biohazard sharps containers.		
2. Disposed of all other regulated medical waste in biohazard bags.		
3. Disinfected test area and instruments according to OSHA guidelines.		
4. Sanitized hands after removing gloves.		
Total Points per Column		

Patient Name: _____

Patient Chart Entry: (Include when, what, how, why, any additional information, and the signature of the person charting.)

_____

_____

_____

8 Microbiology

VOCABULARY REVIEW

Match each definition with the correct term.

_____ 1. Rate at which illness occurs

_____ 2. Having the pink or red color of the counterstain used in Gram's method of staining microorganisms

_____ 3. Diffuse muscle pain

_____ 4. Pertaining to unicellular organisms that do not have a true nucleus with a nuclear membrane

_____ 5. Retaining the purple color of the stain used in Gram's method of staining microorganisms

_____ 6. Disease in the body caused by the invasion of pathogenic microorganisms

_____ 7. Coughing up sputum and mucus from the trachea and lungs

_____ 8. Component made of polysaccharides and peptides that gives rigidity to the bacterial cell wall

_____ 9. Feeling of weakness, distress, or discomfort

_____ 10. Requiring special nutrients for growth

_____ 11. Pertaining to organisms that possess a true nucleus with a nuclear membrane and organelles

_____ 12. Rate of deaths

_____ 13. Asexual reproduction in which the cell splits in half

_____ 14. Mucus expelled from the lungs

_____ 15. Identification of antibiotic of choice to treat an infection

_____ 16. Capable of forming pus

A. malaise
B. myalgia
C. expectoration
D. gram positive
E. fastidious
F. mortality
G. gram negative
H. infection
I. peptidoglycan
J. morbidity
K. eukaryotic
L. prokaryote
M. binary fission
N. sensitivity test
O. purulent
P. sputum

FUNDAMENTAL CONCEPTS

17. Give an example of an organism that is normal flora, and discuss what can occur if the organism is destroyed.

_____

_____

18. Using Table 8-1 in the textbook, list two health issues of concern in the 1990s.

_____

_____

19. List two characteristics of bacteria.

_____

_____

20. Explain the difference between a yeast fungus and a mold fungus.

_____

_____

21. List the three general types of bacterial shapes, and give an example of each.

_____

_____

22. Match each bacterial shape or group with its name (see Figure 8-1 in the textbook).

_____   A. Bacilli

_____   B. Spirilla

_____   C. Streptococci

_____   D. Staphylococci

_____   E. Diplococci

23. Describe the benefits that flagella, spores, and capsules give to organisms that possess these structures.

_____

_____

_____

24. List four ways that medical assistants can take precautions to prevent the spread of infection to others or to themselves.

_____

_____

25. When is the ideal time to collect a microbiology specimen?

_____

_____

26. Discuss the Jembec transport system.

_____

_____

164

27. Describe the cell wall structures that cause some organisms to be gram positive or gram negative.

_____

_____

28. Give the color of gram-positive and gram-negative organisms after the decolorizer step has been applied.

_____

_____

29. Label the supplies needed for Gram staining (see Procedure 8-2 in the textbook).

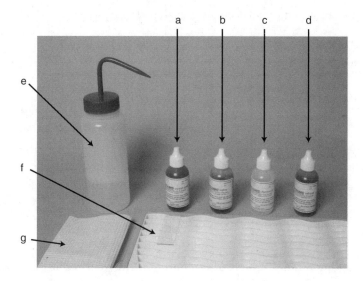

30. What is the causative agent for tuberculosis?

_____

_____

31. Describe the appearance and characteristics of *Trichomonas vaginalis*.

_____

_____

_____

32. Case study: On each blank, write **C** if the statement is correct and **I** if the statement is incorrect. If the step is incorrect, explain why in the space provided.
    A medical assistant is performing Gram staining of a specimen.

_____ 1. The specimen is heat fixed to fix the specimen to the slide.

_____

_____ 2. Crystal violet is applied to the slide for 2 minutes and then rinsed with water.

_____

_____ 3. Gram's iodine is applied for 1 minute, and both gram-positive and gram-negative organisms are purple. Rinse with water.

_____

_____ 4. The decolorizer is applied until the purple has stopped running off the slide. This is the most critical step. Rinse with water.

_____

_____ 5. Safranin is applied last for 1 minute and rinsed with water. Gram-positive organisms are pink or red, and gram-negative organisms are purple.

_____

PROCEDURES: CLINICAL LABORATORY IMPROVEMENT AMENDMENT (CLIA)–WAIVED MICROBIOLOGY TESTS

33. Describe the appearance of alpha, beta, and gamma hemolysis on blood agar plates.

_____

_____

_____

34. State the causative agent (genus and species) of strep throat, and give the most common hemolytic reaction that this organism produces on blood agar plates.

_____

_____

_____

35. What antibiotic is in the disk that is used to identify *Streptococcus pyogenes*?

_____

36. Label the supplies needed to perform a group A *Streptococcus* test (see Procedure 8-5 in the textbook).

37. List three medical conditions associated with a strep infection.

_____

_____

_____

38. When discussing influenza, what is the difference between antigenic *drift* and *shift*?

_____

_____

_____

39. Describe how to obtain a nasal swab specimen when testing for influenza.

_____

_____

ADVANCED CONCEPTS

40. Give the oxygen requirements for aerobic and anaerobic organisms.

_____

_____

41. Name media requirements that most bacteria need for growth.

_____

_____

42. Give the advantages of using an incinerator instead of a Bunsen burner.

_____

_____

43. Describe or draw a picture of the differences between quadrant streaking and colony count streaking.

_____

_____

44. Explain a physician's reason for ordering a sensitivity test.

_____

_____

45. List three organisms that frequently cause urinary tract infections.

_____

_____

46. Case study: Refer to the text section "Pathogenic Organisms Seen Frequently in Physician Office Laboratories" and use Tables 8-4 through 8-9 in the textbook to complete the following information regarding common pathogenic bacteria:

Streptococcus pneumoniae

- Gram stain reaction: _____
- Disease: _____
- Transmission: _____
- Specimens: _____

Neisseria gonorrhoeae

- Gram stain reaction: _____
- Disease: _____
- Transmission: _____
- Specimens: _____

Chlamydia trachomatis

- Disease: _____
- Transmission: _____
- Specimens: _____

Enterobius vermicularis

- Transmission: _____
- Specimens or tests: _____

Urinary tract infections

- Organisms: _____
- Gram stain reaction: _____
- Transmission: _____
- Tests or specimen: _____

Food poisoning (most common cause in the United States)

- Organisms: _____
- Gram stain reaction: _____
- Transmission: _____
- Tests or specimen: _____

Procedure 8-1: Procedure for Collecting a Throat Specimen

Person evaluated _____ Date _____

Evaluated by _____ Score/Grade _____

Outcome goal	To perform throat specimen collection
Conditions	Supplies required: - Sterile swabs and tongue depressor - Personal protective equipment
Standards	Required time: 10 minutes Performance time: _____ Total possible points = _____ Points earned = _____

Evaluation Rubric Codes:
S = Satisfactory, meets standard   **U** = Unsatisfactory, fails to meet standard

NOTE: Steps marked with an asterisk (*) are critical to achieve required competency.

Preparation	Scores	
	S	U
*1. Identified patient and placed in proper position.		
- Had patient state name.		
- Confirmed identification with patient.		
- Compared with requisition.		

Procedure	Scores	
	S	U
*2. Sanitized hands and put on gloves and face mask		
*3. Aseptically removed the sterile Dacron swab (cotton swab may inhibit growth of bacteria) from the package, holding only the tip of the swab.		
4. Had the patient sit with head back.		
*5. Used a sterile tongue depressor to hold down the tongue and had patient say "ahh."		
*6. Rotated the swab on the back of throat in a circular motion or figure-eight pattern.		
- Did not touch the teeth or back of the tongue because these areas have normal flora.		
- Two swabs can be used at the same time: one for a rapid strep test and one for a culture if needed.		
7. Inserted swab into appropriate container for testing.		

Chapter **8** **Microbiology**

8-1

Follow-up	Scores	
	S	**U**
8. Determined if patient was feeling well before dismissing.		
*9. Completed proper documentation on patient chart (see below).		
*10. Proper disposal and disinfection.		
- Disinfected test area and instruments according to OSHA guidelines.		
- Disposed of regulated medical waste (e.g., gloves, tongue depressor) in biohazard bags.		
*11. Sanitized hands.		
Total Points per Column		

Patient Name: _____

Patient Chart Entry: (Include when, what, why, how, any additional information, and the signature of the person charting.)

_____

_____

_____

Procedure 8-2: Gram Stain Procedure

Person evaluated _____   Date _____

Evaluated by _____   Score/Grade _____

Outcome goal	Perform a Gram stain
Conditions	Supplies required: - Gloves, bibulous paper, water bottle or running water - Gram staining reagents: crystal violet, Gram's iodine, decolorizer, safranin - Staining rack
Standards	Required time: 15 minutes Performance time: _____ Total possible points = _____ Points earned = _____ Accuracy = final slide shows gram-positive and gram-negative bacteria

Evaluation Rubric Codes:
S = Satisfactory, meets standard   **U** = Unsatisfactory, fails to meet standard

NOTE: Steps marked with an asterisk (*) are critical to achieve required competency.

Preparation	Scores	
	S	**U**
*1. Sanitized hands and applied gloves.		
*2. Fixed specimen to the slide (using heat or methanol).		
Procedure	**Scores**	
	S	**U**
*3. Applied crystal violet to slide for 1 minute.		
4. Rinsed slide with water.		
*5. Applied Gram's iodine to slide for 1 minute.		
6. Rinsed slide with water.		
*7. Poured decolorizer over the tilted slide until no more purple ran off (about 3 to 5 seconds), and then immediately rinsed slide with water to stop the reaction.		
*8. Applied safranin stain for 1 minute.		
9. Rinsed slide with water.		
10. Blotted slide dry in absorbent bibulous paper.		
Follow-up	**Scores**	
	S	**U**
*11. Proper disposal and disinfection.		
- Disinfected test area and instruments according to OSHA guidelines.		
- Disposed of regulated medical waste (e.g., gloves) in biohazard bags.		
- Sanitized hands.		
Totals Points per Column		

8-2

Patient Name: _____

Patient Chart Entry:

_____

_____

_____

Procedure 8-5: Acceava Strep A Test Procedure

Person evaluated _____ Date _____

Evaluated by _____ Score/Grade _____

Outcome goal	To perform FDA-approved, CLIA-waived rapid strep test following the most current OSHA safety guidelines and applying the correct quality control

Conditions	Supplies required:
	- Acceava rapid strep kit containing:
	  - Reagent 1 and reagent 2
	  - Liquid controls, positive and negative
	  - Soft plastic testing tubes
	  - Test stick and its container
	- Sterile rayon swab taken from wrapper
	- Sterile tongue depressor
	- Gloves, face protection

Standards	Required time: 10 minutes Performance time: _____ Total possible points = _____ Points earned = _____

Evaluation Rubric Codes:
S = Satisfactory, meets standard   **U** = Unsatisfactory, fails to meet standard

NOTE: Steps marked with an asterisk (*) are critical to achieve required competency.

Preparation: Preanalytical Phase	Scores	
	S	**U**
A. Test information		
- Kit or instrument method: **Strep A Test**		
- Manufacturer: **Acceava**		
- Proper storage (e.g., temperature, light): **room temperature**		
- Lot # of kit: _____		
- Expiration date: _____		
- Package insert or test flow chart available: _____ yes _____ no		
B. Specimen information		
- Type of specimen: **throat swab using swab from kit (do not use cotton swabs)**		
C. Personal protective equipment: **gloves, facemask during throat swab, and biohazard container**		

Procedure: Analytical Phase	Scores	
	S	**U**
D. Performed/observed qualitative quality control		
- External liquid controls: positive _____ negative _____		
- Internal control: _____ (appears as a red line on test stick)		
E. Performed patient test		
1. Sanitized hands and applied gloves.		
2. Just before testing, added 3 drops of reagent 1 and 3 drops of reagent 2 into the test tube. The solution should turn light yellow.		

Chapter **8** **Microbiology**

	Scores	
	S	**U**
3. Immediately put the throat swab into the extract solution.		
4. Vigorously mixed the solution by rotating the swab forcefully against the side of the tube at least 10 times. Best results are obtained when the specimen is vigorously extracted in the solution.		
5. Let stand for 1 minute, and then squeezed the swab with the sides of the tube as the swab was withdrawn; discarded the swab into a biohazard container.		
6. Removed a test stick from the container and recapped immediately; placed the absorbent end of the test stick into the extracted sample in the tube.		
7. At 5 minutes, read and recorded the results.		
- Positive = a blue line in test area and pink line in control area, indicating the internal control worked.		
- Negative = no blue line in the test area and a pink line in control area, indicating the internal control worked.		
*Accurate Results _____ Instructor Confirmation _____		

Follow-up: Postanalytical Phase	Scores	
	S	**U**
*F. Proper documentation		
1. On control/patient log: _____ yes _____ no		
2. Documented on patient chart (see below).		
3. Identified critical values and took appropriate steps to notify physician.		
- Expected values for analyte: negative for strep.		
G. Proper disposal and disinfection		
1. Disposed of all sharps in biohazard sharps containers.		
2. Disposed of all other regulated medical waste in biohazard bags.		
3. Disinfected test area and instruments according to OSHA guidelines.		
4. Sanitized hands after removing gloves.		
Totals Points per Column		

Patient Name: _____

Patient Chart Entry: (Include when, what, how, why, any additional information, and the signature of the person charting.)

_____

_____

_____

Procedure 8-6: OSOM Influenza A&B Test Procedure

Person evaluated _____ Date _____

Evaluated by _____ Score/Grade _____

Outcome goal	To perform FDA-approved CLIA-waived influenza test following the most current OSHA safety guidelines and applying the correct quality control
Conditions	Supplies required for the OSOM Influenza A&B Test: - Personal protective equipment (face mask and gloves) - Foam swab provided in kit to collect nasal specimen - Plastic testing tube provided in kit - Extract solution provided in kit - Testing strip provided in kit - Control swabs for influenza A and B - Container of testing strips with diagram showing how to interpret results
Standards	Required time: 10 minutes Performance time: _____ Total possible points = _____ Points earned = _____
Evaluation Rubric Codes: **S** = Satisfactory, meets standard **U** = Unsatisfactory, fails to meet standard	
NOTE: Steps marked with an asterisk (*) are critical to achieve required competency.	

Preparation: Preanalytical Phase	Scores	
	S	**U**
A. Test information		
- Kit or instrument method: **OSOM A&B Influenza Test**		
- Manufacturer: **Genzyme**		
- Proper storage (e.g., temperature, light): **room temperature**		
- Lot # of kit: _____		
- Expiration date: _____		
- Package insert or test flow chart available: _____ yes _____ no		
B. Specimen information		
- Type of specimen: **nasal swab using swab from kit**		
- **Sanitize hands and apply gloves and face mask**		
- Insert the foam swab provided in the test kit into the patient's nostril displaying the most secretion. Using a gentle rotation, push the swab until resistance is met at the level of the turbinates (at least 1 inch into the nostril). Rotate the swab a few times against the nasal wall, and gently rock it back and forth. Hold swab in place for 5 seconds to ensure maximum absorbency.		
C. Personal protective equipment: gloves during testing		

Procedure: Analytical Phase	Scores	
	S	**U**
D. Performed/observed qualitative quality control		
- External swab controls: Positive A _____ Positive B _____		
Negative A _____ Negative B _____		
- Internal control appears as a blue line on test stick.		

E. Performed patient test		
1. Sanitized hands and applied gloves.		
2. Placed the nasal swab into the plastic tube containing the designated amount of extraction buffer solution.		
3. Vigorously twisted the swab against the sides and bottom of the tube at least 10 times, which disrupted the virus particles and released the internal viral nucleoproteins into the solution.		
4. Extracted all the solution from the swab by squeezing the plastic tube against the swab while removing it from the tube and disposed of swab properly.		
5. Dipped the influenza test strip into the tube with the extraction buffer, making sure the arrows on the strip were pointing down.		
6. Allowed 10 minutes for migration of the solution across the test area and control area of the strip, which allowed the nucleoproteins from the virus to react with the reagents on the test strip, causing a color reaction.		
7. Read the results for the influenza A and B test.		
- Positive = Result showed a pink or purple line in the A or B test area and a pink line in the internal control area.		
- Negative = Result showed no color change in the A or B test area and a pink line in the internal control area.		

*Accurate Results _____   **Instructor Confirmation** _____

Follow-up: Postanalytical Phase	Scores	
	S	**U**
*F. Proper documentation		
1. On control/patient log: _____ yes _____ no		
2. Documented on patient chart (see below).		
3. Identified critical values and took appropriate steps to notify physician.		
- Expected values for analyte: negative for influenza A and B.		
G. Proper disposal and disinfection		
1. Disposed of all sharps in biohazard sharps containers.		
2. Disposed of all other regulated medical waste in biohazard bags.		
3. Disinfected test area and instruments according to OSHA guidelines.		
4. Sanitized hands after removing gloves.		
Totals Counts per Column		

Patient Name: _____

Patient Chart Entry: (Include when, what, how, why, any additional information, and the signature of the person charting.)

_____

_____

_____

Procedure 8-7: Rapid Urine Culture Test

Person evaluated _____ Date _____

Evaluated by _____ Score/Grade _____

Outcome goal	To perform FDA-approved CLIA-moderate complexity **Rapid Urine Culture Test** following the most current OSHA safety guidelines and applying the correct quality control
Conditions	**Equipment and Supplies** - Clinical incubator - Uricult kit containing vial with agar-coated slide and reference chart - Gloves - Requisition
Standards	Required time: overnight incubation (18 to 24 hours) Performance time: _____ Total possible points = _____ Points earned = _____

Evaluation Rubric Codes:
S = Satisfactory, meets standard **U** = Unsatisfactory, fails to meet standard

NOTE: Steps marked with an asterisk (*) are critical to achieve required competency.

Preparation: Preanalytical Phase	Scores	
	S	**U**
A. Test information		
- Kit or instrument method: **Uricult**		
- Manufacturer: **LifeSign**		
- Proper storage (e.g., temperature, light): **room temperature**		
- Lot # of kit: _____		
- Expiration date: _____		
- Package insert or test flow chart available: _____ yes _____ no		
B. Specimen information: Have the patient produce a freshly voided clean-catch midstream urine sample that has been in the bladder for a minimum of 4 to 6 hours in the appropriate container. Be sure to mix the urine sample before testing.		
C. Daily monitoring and logging of incubator temperature must be documented.		
D. Personal protective equipment: gloves and gown during testing		

Procedure: Analytical Phase	Scores	
	S	**U**
E. **Quality Control:** No quality control testing required. Visually inspect Uricult vials for contamination, excess moisture, and damage before use. Remove Certificate of Analysis from package insert and document. No standard proficiency survey is required, but the office must participate in a biannual assessment program.		
F. Perform the urine culture test		
1. Unscrew the agar-coated slide from the vial being careful not to touch the agar.		
2. Completely immerse the slide into the urine making sure the agar on both sides of the slide is not immersed for more than several seconds. (Note: If the urine volume in the cup is too small to dip, the urine may be poured over the agar surfaces.)		

	Scores	
	S	U
3. Place the urine-dipped specimen back into the vial and screw the cap on loosely. Label the vial with the patient's name, date, time, and your initials. Place in the incubator.		
4. Read results using reference chart supplied in kit after 18 to 24 hours of incubation (do not exceed 24 hours) (results are interpreted as follows): - *Normal:* Color that reads as <10,000 bacteria/mL of urine indicates the absence of infection. - *Borderline:* Color that reads 10,000 to 100,000 bacteria/mL of urine may indicate a chronic or relapsing infection; it is recommended that the test be repeated. - *Positive:* Color that reads >100,000 bacteria/mL of urine showing complete coverage of the agar surface with bacterial colonies.		
5. Replace the agar slide in the vial and discard in a biohazard bag. Disinfect test area and instruments according to OSHA guidelines.		
*Accurate Results _____ Instructor Confirmation _____		

	Scores	
Follow-up: Postanalytical Phase	S	U
6. Remove the gloves, and sanitize your hands.		
*G. Proper Documentation		
1. On control/patient log: _____ yes _____ no		
2. Documented on patient chart (see below).		
3. Identified critical values and took appropriate steps to notify physician.		
- Expected values for analyte: negative for bacterial infection.		
Totals Points per Column		

Patient Name: _____

Patient Chart Entry: (Include when, what, why, how, any additional information, and the signature of the person charting.)

_____

_____

_____

9 Toxicology

VOCABULARY REVIEW

Match each definition with the correct term.

_____ 1. Methadone and morphine

_____ 2. Blood carrying the drug through the body

_____ 3. Measurement that determines if a substance is present or absent

_____ 4. Abnormal susceptibility to a drug or other agent that is peculiar to the individual

_____ 5. Release of a prescribed drug from its dosage

_____ 6. Level at which a drug becomes poisonous in the body

_____ 7. Precise measurement of the amount of a substance present in the specimen

_____ 8. Marijuana drug screening

_____ 9. Passage of a substance through the surface of the body into body fluids and tissues

_____ 10. FDA-approved drug for treating opioid drug addiction

_____ 11. Movement of drugs through the body from the time of introduction to elimination

_____ 12. Substance produced by the metabolism of a drug in the body

A. idiosyncrasy
B. pharmacokinetics
C. opiates
D. toxicity
E. qualitative drug screening
F. absorption
G. liberation
H. quantitative
I. buprenorphine
J. distribution
K. cannabinoid
L. metabolite

FUNDAMENTAL CONCEPTS

13. List three reasons a specimen would be tested in a toxicology laboratory.

_____

_____

_____

14. List three toxicology responsibilities in the ambulatory care setting.

_____

_____

_____

15. Explain three ways an over-the-counter (OTC) drug can become toxic.

_____

_____

_____

16. Define what makes a drug of abuse.

_____

_____

17. When testing for a drug, urine is usually used for a _____ result, and blood is used for a

_____ result.

18. Describe the *chain of custody* when processing a specimen for drug screening.

_____

_____

19. Define MRO.

_____

_____

20. Explain the results in the urine drug test illustration.

COC _____

AMP _____

mAMP _____

21. Using Table 9-1, write the drug name that matches the following testing codes:

THC _____

COC _____

BUP _____

OPI _____

BAR _____

BZO _____

MTD _____

AMP _____

OXY _____

mAMP _____

22. Why is it important to monitor drug levels during drug therapy?

_____

_____

23. From Table 9-4, list the six drug categories that require therapeutic monitoring.

_____

_____

24. Place the following pharmacokinetic stages in order: metabolism, absorption, liberation, elimination, and distribution.

_____

_____

25. Describe drug *half-life*.

_____

26. List three environmental poisons that are tested in toxicology.

_____

_____

_____

Procedure 9-1: Assisting with Urine Collection for Drug Screening

Person evaluated _____ Date _____

Evaluated by _____ Score/Grade _____

Outcome goal	To assist with urine collection for drug screening
Conditions	Supplies required: - Urine drug screening collection kit with specimen cup with temperature indicator - Urine specimen containers to be sent to the laboratory - Plastic sealable pouch for the two urine specimen containers, chain of custody documents - Personal protective equipment
Standards	Required time: 15 minutes Performance time: _____ Total possible points = _____ Points earned = _____
Evaluation Rubric Codes: **S** = Satisfactory, meets standard **U** = Unsatisfactory, fails to meet standard	
NOTE: Steps marked with an asterisk (*) are critical to achieve required competency.	

Preparation	Scores	
	S	**U**
1. Explain to the patient the purpose of the test and the procedure to be followed for a midstream clean-catch specimen collection.		
- Had patient state name.		
- Obtained a signed consent form from the patient.		
- Compared with requisition.		

Procedure	Scores	
	S	**U**
2. Sanitized hands and put on gloves and face mask.		
3. A trained professional must witness the voiding of at least 50 mL of urine into the specimen cup provided in the urine collection drug kit.		
4. Originate the chain of custody document at the time of the sample collection. The person who witnessed the voiding must sign the document, as must every other person who handles the sample.		
5. After the collection, verify the temperature of the urine as seen on the indicator at the bottom of the cup, and document it. *Note:* If the temperature of the urine specimen is out of range (too cold), a second specimen must be collected. If the donor refuses to provide the second specimen under direct observation, the collection would be considered a "refusal to test."		
*6. Transfer the specimen to the two containers that must be labeled with the following information: - Full name of the patient - Date and time of collection - Your initials - Initials of the witnessing officer		
7. Place the two sample containers into the sealed plastic pouch, mark it with a notary-style seal or with tamper-proof tape to protect the integrity of the sample, and send the specimen to the toxicology laboratory.		

8. If you are trained and qualified to do the testing, proceed with the testing according to laboratory and state regulations.		
Follow-up	**Scores**	
	S	**U**
9. After the initial and confirmatory testing is complete, mark the urine sample, reseal it, and securely store it for a minimum of 30 days or for the length of time specified by laboratory protocols.		
10. Completed proper documentation on patient chart (see below).		
11. Proper disposal and disinfection.		
- Disinfected test area and instruments according to OSHA guidelines.		
- Disposed of regulated medical waste (e.g., gloves, tongue depressor) in biohazard bags.		
*12. Sanitized hands.		
Total Points per Column		

Patient Name: _____

Patient Chart Entry: (Include when, what, how, why, any additional information, and the signature of the person charting.)

_____

_____

_____

Procedure 9-2: Assisting with Blood Collection for Alcohol Testing

Person evaluated _____ Date _____

Evaluated by _____ Score/Grade _____

Outcome goal	To assist with blood collection for drug screening
Conditions	Supplies required: - Gray-topped Vacutainer tubes - Venipuncture needle and holder (or syringe and transfer device) - Nonvolatile disinfectant (e.g., benzalkonium [Zephiran], aqueous thimerosal [Merthiolate]) - Gauze - Tourniquet - Gloves - Legally authorized transportation envelope, container, or plastic pouch
Standards	Required time: 15 minutes Performance time: _____ Total possible points = _____ Points earned = _____
Evaluation Rubric Codes: **S** = Satisfactory, meets standard **U** = Unsatisfactory, fails to meet standard	
NOTE: Steps marked with an asterisk (*) are critical to achieve required competency.	

Patient Preparation	Scores	
	S	**U**
1. An officer of the law is present to act as a witness to the procedure.		
2. The patient probably is likely still to be under the influence of alcohol, so explain what you will be doing in as concise a manner as possible. *Note:* Do not allow yourself to become irritated by the speech or mannerisms of the patient. Treat the patient with the respect and dignity with which you treat all patients.		

Blood Collection Procedure	Scores	
	S	**U**
Note: The Department of Justice for each state has established uniform standards for the collection, handling, and preservation of blood samples used for alcohol testing. If you are authorized to obtain specimens for forensic analysis, check your laboratory's procedure manual so that you perform the collection *exactly* as required by the uniform standards established for your state.		
3. Sanitize hands, and apply gloves.		
4. Prepare the draw site using Zephiran, aqueous Merthiolate, or another aqueous disinfectant. *Do not use alcohol or other volatile organic disinfectants to clean the skin site.*		
5. Complete the blood draw, filling both tubes with sufficient blood to permit duplicate blood alcohol determinations.		
6. Label the two gray-stoppered tubes with the following information: - Full name of the patient - Date and time of collection - Your initials - Initials of the witnessing officer		

7. Give the labeled blood samples to the witnessing officer, who will immediately complete the required information on the transportation envelope, container, or plastic pouch. The officer will then seal it securely. Information on the envelope or container should include the following: - The full name of the patient - Whether the patient is alive or dead - The submitting agency - The geographic location where the blood was drawn (e.g., hospital, clinic, jail) - The name of the person drawing the blood sample - The date and time the blood sample was drawn - The signature of the witnessing officer		
8. After the envelope or container is sealed, it must not be opened except for analysis. Each person who is subsequently in possession of the sealed sample must sign his or her name in the space provided on the envelope or container (chain of custody). The integrity of the sample must be safeguarded.		
9. Remove gloves, and wash hands.		
Total Points per Column		

Patient Name: _____

Patient Chart Entry: (Include when, what, how, why, any additional information, and the signature of the person charting.)

_____

_____

_____

Procedure 9-3: Urine Drug Panel Testing Procedure

Person evaluated _____ Date _____

Evaluated by _____ Score/Grade _____

Outcome goal	To perform FDA-approved, CLIA-waived drug panel test following the most current OSHA safety guidelines and applying the correct quality control
Conditions	Supplies required: - Gloves - Test card with multiple test strips (five tests are on each side of the card) - Metal pouch containing test card that has been stored at 2° C to 30° C (check expiration date)
Standards	Required time: 10 minutes Performance time: _____ Total possible points = _____ Points earned = _____

Evaluation Rubric Codes:
S = Satisfactory, meets standard   **U** = Unsatisfactory, fails to meet standard

NOTE: Steps marked with an asterisk (*) are critical to achieve required competency.

Preparation: Preanalytical Phase	Scores	
	S	**U**
A. Test information		
- Kit method:		
- Manufacturer:		
- Proper storage (e.g., temperature, light): store the card at 2° C to 30° C (check expiration date)		
- Lot # of kit: _____		
- Expiration date: _____		
- Package insert or test flow chart available: _____ yes _____ no		
B. Specimen information		
- Type of specimen: **Fresh urine specimen or specimen that has been stored at 2° C to 8° C for up to 48 hours and then brought to room temperature.**		
C. Sanitize the hands, and apply gloves.		

Procedure: Analytical Phase	Scores	
	S	**U**
D. Performed/observed qualitative quality control		
- External liquid controls: positive _____ negative _____		
- Internal control: _____ (appears as a red line on test stick)		
E. Performed patient test		
1. Sanitize the hands, and apply gloves.		
2. Remove the test device from its protective pouch, and label it with the patient's identification. *Note*: If the specimen has been stored in the refrigerator, bring it to room temperature before opening to prevent condensation.		
3. Remove the cap from the end of the test card.		

	Scores	
	S	**U**

4. With the arrows pointing toward the urine specimen, immerse the strips of the test card vertically into the urine specimen for at least 10 to 15 seconds. **Immerse the strips to at least the level of the wavy lines on the strips but not above the arrows on the test card.**

5. Place the test card on a nonabsorbent surface, and wait for the colored lines to appear.

6. At 5 minutes, read and record the results.

- Positive test result: One distinct pink band appears in the control region (C), with no line in the test region (T).

- Negative test result: Two pink bands appear, with one pink band in the control region (C) and one pink band in the patient test region (T).

- Invalid: Pink bands are absent from the control region. Repeat the test with a new device. If the problem persists, call for technical assistance.

*Accurate Results _____ Instructor Confirmation _____

Follow-up: Postanalytical Phase	Scores	
	S	**U**
*F. Proper documentation		
1. On control/patient log: _____ yes _____ no		
2. Documented on patient chart (see below).		
3. Identified critical values and took appropriate steps to notify physician.		
- Expected values for analytes: negative		
G. Proper disposal and disinfection		
1. Disposed of all sharps in biohazard sharps containers.		
2. Disposed of all other regulated medical waste in biohazard bags.		
3. Disinfected test area and instruments according to OSHA guidelines.		
4. Sanitized hands after removing gloves.		
Total Points per Column		

Patient Name: _____

Patient Chart Entry: (Include when, what, how, why, any additional information, and the signature of the person charting.)

_____

_____

_____

10 Electrocardiography and Spirometry

VOCABULARY REVIEW

Match each definition with the correct term.

Cardiology Terms

_____ 1. The relaxation phase in the heart when there is no electrical activity within the cardiac muscle

_____ 2. Pattern of P, Q, R, S, T, and U waves on an ECG recording

_____ 3. Pump the blood out of the heart to the lungs and the body

_____ 4. 12 ECG recordings that consist of 6 limb leads and 6 chest leads

_____ 5. The 10 "sensors" placed on the limbs and chest that detect the electrical activity of the heart

_____ 6. Tracings other than from the heart or lungs that interfere with the interpretation of the ECG or spirometer recordings

_____ 7. Rapid irregular contraction of a muscle

_____ 8. Fast heart rate

_____ 9. Receive blood from the body on the right side and from the lungs on the left side

_____ 10. The contraction phase of the heart when the cardiac muscle is being stimulated by electrical impulses

_____ 11. Sends out an electrical impulse that starts the heartbeat

_____ 12. A sequence of two cardiac phases: a contraction phase and a relaxation phase

_____ 13. A muscular wall that divides the right and left sides of the heart

_____ 14. Heart rhythm is within normal limits

_____ 15. Blood flowing to the body and back to the heart

_____ 16. Slow heart rate

_____ 17. When the atria or ventricles contract prematurely

A. bradycardia
B. fibrillation
C. systole
D. atria
E. ECG cycle
F. systemic circulation
G. ECG leads
H. septum
I. artifacts
J. cardiac cycle
K. diastole
L. electrodes
M. sinus rhythm
N. premature contractions
O. tachycardia
P. sinoatrial (SA) node
Q. ventricles

Skeletal and Pulmonary Terms

_____ 18. Breast bone

_____ 19. Forced vital capacity—amount of air exhaled in 6 seconds

_____ 20. Measurement of the volume and flow of air that is breathed

_____ 21. Chronic obstructive pulmonary disease

_____ 22. Between the ribs

_____ 23. Blood flowing to the lungs and back to the heart

_____ 24. Collar bone

A. intercostal
B. pulmonary circulation
C. FVC
D. spirometry
E. sternum
F. peak flow rate
G. artifacts
H. COPD
I. FEV_1
J. clavicle

189

_____ 25. Tracings other than from the heart or lungs that interfere with the interpretation of the ECG or spirometer recordings

_____ 26. A test that measures how fast a person can exhale

_____ 27. Forced expiratory volume in the first second expressed in liters

FUNDAMENTAL CONCEPTS

Heart Anatomy and the ECG

28. Blood enters the right and left _____ of the heart, and is pumped out of the heart by the right and left _____.

29. The cardiac cycle consists of a contraction phase known as _____ and a relaxation phase known as _____.

30. Identify the five electrical conduction structures in the heart and the heart chambers that contract as a result of electrical stimulation (see Figure 10-3 in text).

31. Who invented the first practical electrocardiogram? _____ What were his first three "leads" or tracings of the heart beating? _____. Each of these leads required two limbs and were referred to as _____ leads.

32. How many electrodes are used in the standard ECG? _____ How many leads are recorded? _____

33. Label the nine components involved in recording an ECG tracing. (Note: Refer to Figure 10-8 in text.)

34. Match the following leads with their approptiate electrical descriptors:

_____ and _____ and _____ V$_1$, V$_2$, V$_3$, V$_4$, V$_5$, and V$_6$ A. Augmented limb leads

_____ and _____ I, II, and III   B. Unipolar leads (used twice)

_____ and _____ aVR, aVF, and aVL   C. Standard limb leads

                                                                         D. Chest leads

                                                                         E. Bipolar leads

                                                                         F. Precordial leads

35. Match the chest leads with their appropriate electrode placement

_____ V1	A. Midway between the V2 and V4 positions
_____ V2	B. 4th intercostal space on the left side of the sternum leads
_____ V3	C. 5th intercostal space on the left midclavicular line
_____ V4	D. Horizontal to V4 at the left midaxillary line
_____ V5	E. Horizontal to V4 at the left anterior axillary line
_____ V6	F. 4th intercostal space on the right side of the patient's sternum

36. Draw a standard pulse and one ECG tracing. Then label the waves: P, Q, R, S, and T. (Refer to Figure 10-11 in the text.)

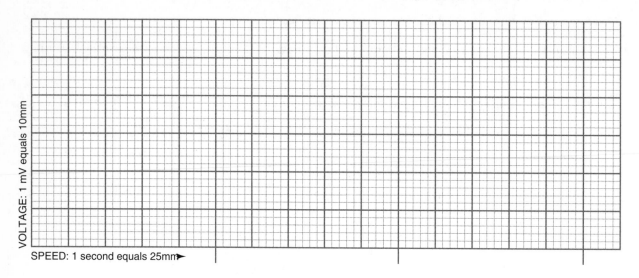

VOLTAGE: 1 mV equals 10mm

SPEED: 1 second equals 25mm

Anatomy of the Lungs and Spirometry

37. Match the following respiratory structures with their anatomical descriptions (A-D) and their associated obstructive disease descriptions (E-H):

Terminal bronchioles: _____ and _____	A. Primary, secondary, and tertiary bronchi
	B. Air sacs where gas exchanges take place
Lower respiratory tract: _____ and _____	C. Small airways capable of dilating or constricting
	D. Nasal cavity, pharynx, larynx, trachea
Upper respiratory tract: _____ and _____	E. Walls break down most commonly caused by smoking (emphysema)
	F. Infections such as colds, flu, allergies
Alveoli: _____ and _____	G. Muscles become swollen, and thick mucus forms causing difficulty breathing in or out (asthma)
	H. Chronic condition typically caused by smoking, toxic fumes, or other irritants (bronchitis)

38. List the three steps of the spirometry "manuever."

Step 1: _____

Step 2: _____

Step 3: _____

39. Match the "Volume/time chart" and the "Peak flow chart" that are produced during a spirometry test with the results they produce:

Volume/time chart	A. **PEF**—peak expiratory flow
1. _____	B. **FET**—forced expiratory time
2. _____	C. **FEF**$_{25\%-75\%}$
3. _____	D. **FVC**—forced vital capacity
4. _____	E. **FEV**$_1$—forced expiratory volume in the first second
Flow/volume chart—"Peak flow chart"	F. **FEV**$_1$**/FVC ratio**—a healthy person is predicted to exhale 80% to 90% of his or her total volume (FVC) within the first second (FEV$_1$).
1. _____	
2. _____	

40. When calibrating the spirometer, how many liters are sent into the mouthpiece? _____ What are the two enviromental factors that affect the spirometry reading?

_____ and _____

DIAGNOSTIC PROCEDURES

ECG Patient Preparations, Instructions, and Identification of Artifacts

41. Two ways to reduce a patient's anxiety about the ECG test is to refer to it as a _____ test and refer to the sticky electrodes as _____.

42. What should you do if a large patient does not have room on the examination table to rest his arms comfortably?

_____

43. Why should the patient remain still during the ECG recording?

_____

44. Write down the causes (or names) of the four artifacts seen on the ECG tracings below (A-D). And then match each artifact example with two ways to correct the artifact from the answers (a - h) below.

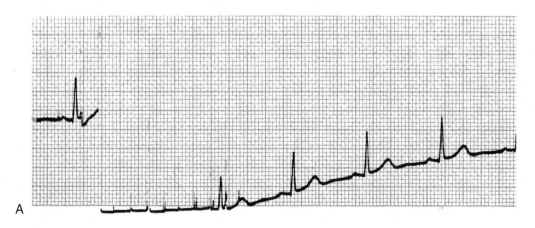

A

(Modified from Bonewit-West K: *Clinical procedures for medical assistants,* ed 9, St Louis, 2015, Saunders, with reference to Long BW: *Radiography essentials for limited practice,* ed 3, 2010, Saunders.)

Continued

Name the 4 artifacts shown above (A - D). Then, match the causes and ways to correct from the answers a. thru h. below. (Note: Each artifact has two corrections from the list of a - h below.)

A. _____ Causes/Corrections: _____ and _____

B. _____ Causes/Corrections: _____ and _____

C. _____ Causes/Corrections: _____ and _____

D. _____ Causes/Corrections: _____ and _____

a. Check if patient is comfortable and relaxed.
b. The electrode is not making contact because of hair on the legs or chest. Shave the site and reapply a new electrode.
c. Check if the patient cable or the lead wires are dangling and not supported.
d. Check if the power cord is running under the examination table.
e. The cable showing the interrupted pattern may be damaged and may need to be replaced.
f. Have the patient hold his or her breath for 15 seconds.
g. The patient has Parkinson's disease with involuntary muscle tremors in the limbs.
h. Check if high-voltage wiring is running parallel in the walls or overhead.

45. While recording the ECG, you see interference in leads II and III but not in lead I. What limb is causing the interference?

_____

Spirometer Patient Preparations, Instructions, and Identification of Artifacts

46. List the three things a patient should do to prepare for a spirometry test.

_____

_____

_____

47. When coaching a patient during spirometry, indicate with a "P" if the feedback statement is positive and an "N" if the feedback statement is negative.

_____	"Keep your eyes on the screen."
_____	"You didn't blow long enough."
_____	"You're not putting the mouthpiece far enough into your mouth."
_____	"I need you to blow out really hard."
_____	"Don't look away."
_____	"You didn't blow hard enough."
_____	"I need you to blow until I say stop."
_____	"I need you to seal you lips firmly around the mouthpiece so all your breath is captured."

48. What can be done to help the patient keep blowing for the full 6 seconds of the manuever?

_____

49. If the patient shows signs of airway obstruction, the physician may order a post-bronchodilator test. Why?

_____

ADVANCED CONCEPTS

Peak Expiratory Flow Screening and Monitoring

50. The manuever for using the ambulatory peak flow monitor (PFM) has only two steps. Describe these steps.

Step 1:

_____

_____

Step 2:

_____

_____

51. When using a peak flow meter in the ambulatory setting, the patient's results are compared with other individuals with the same three demographics. List them.

1. _____

2. _____

3. _____

52. List the symptoms and physical findings seen in a child experiencing an asthmatic attack and respiratory distress.

_____

_____

_____

53. When an asthmatic child is measuring and recording his peak flow meter results daily, it is important to explain the significance of the three colored "zones." Briefly state what each zone represents.

Green zone: _____

Yellow zone: _____

Red zone: _____

54. List the three ways asthmathic patients may find relief when they are experiencing respiratory distress.

1. _____

2. _____

3. _____

55. List the two basic types of drug therapies used in asthma treatment. (Hint: One reduces swelling and mucus formation, and the other relaxes the muscles in the bronchioles.)

_____

_____

56. Describe the difference between a metered dose inhaler and a nebulizer for the delivery of medications.

_____

_____

_____

57. Why should you be familiar with administering nebulizer and oxygen treatments in the ambulatory setting?

_____

_____

Ambulatory ECG Monitoring and Cardiac Pathology and the ECG

58. List two portable ways a patient may monitor his or her ECG over time.

_____

_____

59. Considering all the examples of atrial arrhythmias and ventricular arrhythmias, which is the most serious and life-threatening? Hint: Think of a heart attack that requires cardiopulmonary resuscitation (CPR) using a defibrillator.

_____

Procedure 10-1: Electrocardiography

Person evaluated _____   Date _____

Evaluated by _____   Score/Grade _____

Outcome goal	To demonstrate the proper technique for preparing the patient and recording a diagnostic ECG
Conditions	Given the following supplies: - (Razor) - Alcohol - 10 disposable electrodes - Patient cable with lead wires - Power cord - Gown for the patient - ECG three-channel instrument or computerized ECG program to connect the patient cable
Standards	Required time: 20 minutes Performance time: _____ Total possible points = _____ Points earned = _____

Evaluation Rubric Codes:
S = Satisfactory, meets standard   **U** = Unsatisfactory, fails to meet standard

NOTE: Steps marked with an asterisk (*) are critical to achieve required competency.

Preparation: Preanalytical Phase	Scores	
	S	**U**
A. Test information		
- Burdick three-channel or Midmark computerized program		
- Lot # on disposable electrodes: _____		
- Expiration date on electrode package: _____		
- Instructions provided by ECG manufacturer: _____ yes _____ no		
B. Patient preparation		
1. Cleansed hands and prepared room with clean table paper, pillow, gown, and drape.		
2. Greeted the patient and confirmed identity while entering demographic data (i.e., patient's name, number, age, address). Instructed patient how to apply gown and provided privacy as they disrobed and put on gown.		
3. After returning, obtained the patient's vital signs and entered the vital signs into the computer.		
4. Prepared the 10 sites in the following routine order:		
- Prepare the lower limbs by dry shaving the inner calf muscles if necessary and then rub the areas with an alcohol swab to encourage circulation at the sites.		
- Prepare the upper outer limbs with the alcohol swab followed by locating the general areas for the chest leads and rubbing the areas with the alcohol swab.		
- Return to the legs and arms, and firmly press the electrode sensors with the tabs up on the legs and the tabs down on the arms. Check color-coded lead wires: green on RL, red on LL, black on LA, and white on RA.		

5. Relocated the actual chest sites by palpation and placed the electrodes in the following order:		
- Locate the 4th intercostal space across to the right side of the patient's sternum then place the V_1 **electrode** with the tab down followed by the V_2 **electrode** directly across the sternum on the patient's left side (closest to you).		
- Locate the V_4 lead location by following the 5th intercostal space and the intersecting midclavicular line and place the V_4 **electrode** on the site followed by the V_3 **electrode** midway between V_2 and V_4.		
- Locate the last two lead locations by following a horizontal line around the ribs, based on the location of V_4, and place V_5 **electrode** on the intersecting anterior-lateral line of the chest and V_6 **electrode** at the intersecting midaxillary line of the chest.		
- Methodically connect the numbered V_1–V_6 **lead wires** to each of their designated electrode locations.		

Procedure: Analytical Phase	Scores	
	S	**U**
C. Performed/observed quality control by checking the speed of the paper was set at 25 mm/sec and the 0.1 mV caused a 10-mm rise on the recording.		
D. Performed the electrocardiography.		
1. Before starting the recording, the patient was informed that they needed to be very still and relaxed for about 15 seconds or so while the ECG is monitoring their heartbeats.		
2. Observed the three-channel ECG printout or the computer results for the following:		
- Check each lead in the tracing for unwanted artifacts and correct them if possible (i.e., AC interference, muscle tremors, wandering or interrupted baseline). Re-record another tracing if necessary.		
- Allow the physician to see the final product before disconnecting the patient from the ECG.		
*Accurate Results _____ Instructor Confirmation _____		

Follow-up: Postanalytical Phase	Scores	
	S	**U**
*E. Proper documentation		
1. On control log _____ yes _____ no		
2. On patient log _____ yes _____ no		
3. Documented on patient chart (see below)		
F. Proper disposal and disinfection		
1. Removed and disposed of the electrodes and helped the patient to sitting position.		
2. Instructed the patient to get dressed and that the physician would be sharing the findings with the patient.		
3. Disinfected test area and instruments according to OSHA guidelines.		
4. Sanitized hands.		
Totals Counts per Column		

Patient Name: _____

Patient Chart Entry: (Include when, what, how, why, any additional information, and the signature of the person charting.)

_____

_____

_____

Procedure 10-2: Spirometry

Person evaluated _____ Date _____

Evaluated by _____ Score/Grade _____

Outcome goal	To demonstrate the proper technique for preparing the patient and recording a diagnostic spirometer test
Conditions	Given the following supplies: - Spirometer instrument or computer connected to printers - A disposable sterile mouthpiece connected to the plastic tubing on the spirometer (take care not to touch the area where the patient's mouth will be placed) - A nose clip (based on the physician's preference) - A chair should be available for the patient to sit on if he or she becomes fatigued during the maneuver - Disposable gloves to be worn during and after the patient's test to avoid the transmission of possible respiratory viruses and other respiratory pathogens - 3-liter syringe for calibrating the spirometer
Standards	Required time: 20 minutes Performance time: _____ Total possible points = _____ Points earned = _____

Evaluation Rubric Codes:
S = Satisfactory, meets standard   **U** = Unsatisfactory, fails to meet standard

NOTE: Steps marked with an asterisk (*) are critical to achieve required competency.

Preparation: Preanalytical Phase	Scores	
	S	**U**
A. Test information		
- Midmark computerized spirometer program (or other)		
- Lot # on disposable mouthpiece: _____		
- Instructions provided by ECG manufacturer: _____ yes _____ no		
B. Patient preparation		
1. Called the patient into the room and sanitized hands while confirming the patient's identity by asking for three identifiers: spell last name, give date of birth; and provide one more identifier such as: phone number, address, or driver's license.		
2. Entered the following data into the spirometer: patient's name, ID number, age, height, weight, gender, and race. NOTE: All this information is critical for the spirometer to produce the appropriate "predicted" results.		
3. Confirmed when the patient last took bronchodilator medication and if he or she smoked and noted it on the chart. Also, if appropriate, checked to make sure the patient does not have loose dentures that would interfere with the breathing maneuver.		
4. Explained and demonstrated the three steps of the maneuver using a mouthpiece that is not connected to the spirometer:		
- **Fully inflate** lungs and then held your breath while sealing lips around the mouthpiece.		
- **Fully exhale** into the mouthpiece as fast and as hard as possible.		
- **Give full effort** to exhale the remaining air in lungs for another 5 seconds without inhaling until the time is up.		
5. Showed and explained the importance of standing upright during the maneuver and that the patient will have a minute to rest and sit between a minimum of three attempts.		

199

Chapter **10** **Electrocardiography and Spirometry**

Procedure: Analytical Phase	Scores	
	S	U
C. Performed/observed quality control by running a test using the 3-liter calibration syringe with results falling within + or − 3% of 3 liters.		
D. Performed the spirometer test.		
1. Coached the patient as they performed the maneuver. Watched them making sure they performed all three steps: inspiration, rapid exhalation, and extended exhalation. Praised what they did well and communicated positive ways to improve the next maneuver. Did not give negative feedback.		
2. Observed the two graph results and the spirometer feedback after each maneuver and had the patient rest for a minute:		
- The *time/volume curve* should have shown a sharp rise within the first second and then a slight steady rise for the next 2 to 6 seconds.		
- The *volume/flow curve* should have shown a fast rise in the beginning of the graph with a gradual curve downward that ends on the baseline.		
3. Repeated at least three maneuvers, until the patient was able to perform two reproducible results.		
*Accurate Results _____ Instructor Confirmation _____		

Follow-up: Postanalytical Phase	Scores	
	S	U
*E. Proper documentation		
1. On control log _____ yes _____ no		
2. On patient log _____ yes _____ no		
3. Documented on patient chart (see below)		
F. Proper disposal and disinfection		
1. Discarded the patient's mouthpiece and gloves in biohazard container and sanitized hands.		
2. Instructed the patient to get dressed and that the physician would be sharing the findings with the patient.		
3. Disinfected test area and instruments according to OSHA guidelines.		
Totals Counts per Column		

Patient Name: _____

Patient Chart Entry: (Include when, what, how, why, any additional information, and the signature of the person charting.)

_____

_____

_____

10-2

Procedure 10-3: Peak Expiratory Flow Monitoring

Person evaluated _____ Date _____

Evaluated by _____ Score/Grade _____

Outcome goal	To demonstrate the proper technique for measuring a patient's peak expiratory flow using a peak flow monitor
Conditions	Given the following supplies: - Height/weight scale - New or sterilized peak flow meter - Additional peak flow meter for demonstrating maneuver - Daily monitoring chart
Standards	Required time: 20 minutes Performance time: _____ Total possible points = _____ Points earned = _____

Evaluation Rubric Codes:
S = Satisfactory, meets standard **U** = Unsatisfactory, fails to meet standard

NOTE: Steps marked with an asterisk (*) are critical to achieve required competency.

Preparation: Preanalytical Phase	Scores	
	S	**U**
A. Patient preparation		
1. Called the patient into the room and sanitized your hands while confirming the patient's identity by asking for three identifiers: spell last name, give date of birth: and provide one more identifier such as: phone number, address, or driver's license.		
2. Confirmed when the patient last took bronchodilator medication and if he or she had a heavy meal in the last 4 hours.		
3. Measured patient's height in inches and confirmed patient's age (to compare with proper demographic group if it is a screening test).		
4. Explained and demonstrated the two steps of the maneuver using a demo peak flow meter:		
- **Fully inflate** lungs and then held your breath while sealing lips around the mouthpiece.		
- **Fully exhale** into the mouthpiece as fast and as hard as possible.		
5. Showed and explained the importance of standing upright during the maneuver and that the patient will have a minute to rest and sit between a minimum of three attempts.		

Procedure: Analytical Phase	Scores	
	S	**U**
B. Taught the patient as follows:		
1. Before each use, make sure the sliding pointer on the peak flow meter is reset to the zero mark.		
2. Stand up straight, and remove chewing gum or any food from your mouth.		
3. Take a deep breath and put the mouthpiece in your mouth. Seal your lips and teeth tightly around the mouthpiece.		
4. Record the number where the sliding pointer has stopped on the scale.		
5. Reset the pointer to zero. Repeat this routine three times. You will know you have done the technique correctly when the three readings are close together.		
6. Record the highest of the three readings on a graph or in a notebook. This is called the *"best effort."*		
7. Use the peak flow meter once a day or as directed by your physician. Measure peak flows about the same time each day. A good time might be when you first wake up or at bedtime.		

201

C. Tested the patient as follows		
8. Coached the patient as he or she performed the maneuver. Watched the patient to make sure both steps were performed: inspiration and rapid exhalation. Praised what the patient did well and communicated positive ways to improve the next maneuver. Did not give negative feedback.		
9. **If the patient is taking a screening test:** Located the patient's predicted value on the *Peak Expiratory Flow Rate Table* at the end of this procedure based on age, gender, and height. Divided the predicted value into the patient's result. If less than 80% of the predicted value, patient may need further evaluation.		
10. **If the patient is prescribed daily peak flow monitoring:** Determined the patient's "best effort" reading from three attempts. The personal best value is used as a baseline for routine measurements. Showed the patient the daily peak flow chart at the end of this procedure where the patient will enter daily results. Explain the importance of noting the three colored zones: green = good, yellow = contact the physician, red = danger, seek proper care.		

Quality Control	S	U
D. Made the patient aware of the following issues that prevent accurate readings and how to correct them:		
- Coughing during the maneuver will require the maneuver to be repeated.		
- Poor seal around the mouthpiece while performing the procedure will give false low readings.		
- Taking asthma medication before the peak flow meter (especially bronchodilator medication) will open the airways and give a false high reading.		
- A dirty meter will not record accurately.		
- Blocking the mouthpiece with the tongue will give a false low reading.		
- Using a different type or brand of peak flow meter will cause the measurements to vary among brands and types of meters.		

*Accurate Results _____ Instructor Confirmation _____

Follow-up: Postanalytical Phase	Scores	
	S	U
*E. Proper documentation		
1. On control log _____ yes _____ no		
2. On patient log _____ yes _____ no		
3. Documented on patient chart (see below)		
F. Proper disposal and disinfection		
- Disinfected test area and instruments according to OSHA guidelines.		
Totals Counts per Column		

Patient Name: _____

Patient Chart Entry: (Include when, what, how, why, any additional information, and the signature of the person charting.)

_____

_____

_____

TABLE 10-1: PEAK EXPIRATORY FLOW RATES*

Child and Adolescent Female: 6-20 Years of Age

Height (inches)	42	46	50	54	57	60	64	68	72
Age									
6	134	164	193	223	245	268	297	327	357
8	153	182	212	242	264	287	316	346	376
10	171	201	231	261	283	305	335	365	395
12	190	220	250	280	302	324	354	384	414
14	209	239	269	298	321	343	373	403	432
16	228	258	288	318	340	362	392	421	451
18	247	277	306	336	358	381	411	440	470
20	266	295	325	355	377	400	429	459	489

Child and Adolescent Male: 6-25 Years of Age

Height (inches)	44	48	52	56	60	64	68	72	76
Age									
6	99	146	194	241	289	336	384	431	479
8	119	166	214	261	309	356	404	451	499
10	139	186	234	281	329	376	424	471	519
12	159	206	254	301	349	396	444	491	539
14	178	226	274	321	369	416	464	511	559
16	198	246	293	341	389	436	484	531	579
18	218	266	313	361	408	456	503	551	599
20	238	286	333	381	428	476	523	571	618
22	258	306	353	401	448	496	543	591	638
24	278	326	373	421	468	516	563	611	658
25	288	336	383	431	478	526	573	621	668

Continued

TABLE 10-1: PEAK EXPIRATORY FLOW RATES—cont'd

Adult Female: 20-80 Years of Age

Height (inches)	58	60	62	64	66	68	70		
Age									
20	357	372	387	402	417	432	446		
25	350	365	379	394	409	424	439		
30	342	357	372	387	402	417	431		
35	335	350	364	379	394	409	424		
40	327	342	357	372	387	402	416		
45	320	335	349	364	379	394	409		
50	312	327	342	357	372	387	401		
55	308	320	334	349	364	379	394		
60	297	312	327	342	357	372	386		
65	290	305	319	334	349	364	379		
70	282	297	312	327	342	357	371		
75	275	290	304	319	334	349	364		
80	267	282	297	312	327	342	356		

Adult Male: 25-80 Years of Age

Height (inches)	63	65	67	69	71	73	75	77	
Age: 24	492	520	549	578	606	635	664	692	
30	481	510	538	567	596	624	653	682	
35	471	499	528	557	585	614	643	671	
40	460	489	517	546	575	603	632	661	
45	450	478	507	536	564	593	622	650	
50	439	468	496	525	554	582	611	640	
55	429	457	486	515	543	572	601	629	
60	418	447	475	504	533	561	590	619	
65	408	436	465	494	522	551	580	608	
70	397	426	454	483	512	540	569	598	
75	387	405	444	473	501	530	559	587	
80	376	405	433	462	491	519	5		

From www.sh.lsuhsc.edu/fammed/outpatientmanual/PeakFlowTables.htm. Accessed January 2, 2014.

*Note that the values are the average normal values for healthy persons of a given age and height (Knudson, 1976). There will always be a range of normal values; not everyone can be expected to have exactly the same value. Men can have peak flow values as low as 100 L/min less than the average value shown and still fall within the normal range. Women can have peak flow values as low as 80 L/min less than the average value shown and still fall within the normal range.

PEAK FLOW CHART

Name _____

Week Beginning (date) _____

Peak Flow Zones: Green Zone _____ Yellow Zone _____ Red Zone _____

Prescribed Medications (include dose and frequency) _____

Peak Flow Recording Times: _____ AM _____ PM

DATE	/	/	/	/	/	/	/	/	/	/	/	/	/	/
TIME														
600														
550														
500														
45														
400														
350														
300														
250														
200														
150														
100														
50														
Peak Flow Number														
Notes														

PEAK FLOW CHART

Name _____

Peak Flow Zones: Green Zone _____ Yellow Zone _____ Red Zone _____

Prescribed Medications (include dose and frequency) _____

Peak Flow Recording Times: _____ AM _____ PM

DATE	/	/	/	/	/	/	/	/	/	/	/	/	/	/		
TIME																
600																
550																
500																
45																
400																
350																
300																
250																
200																
150																
100																
50																
Peak Flow Number																
Notes																

Procedure 10-4: Holter Monitoring

Person evaluated _____ Date _____

Evaluated by _____ Score/Grade _____

Outcome goal	To demonstrate the proper technique to prepare a patient for Holter or ambulatory monitoring of ECG over time
Conditions	Given the following supplies: There are a variety of Holter monitoring systems in use. Most systems provide patient packets with all the supplies for preparing the patient included. The Midmark Holter packet consists of the following: - Five white electrodes to be placed on chest landmarks - Sterile razor for removing hair from sites - Abrasive pad to increase circulation at the sites - Alcohol swabs for removing oil and sweat - Patient cable with four lead wires and a green ground wire - New batteries for the monitor - Patient log for recording cardiac "events"
Standards	Required time: 20 minutes Performance time: _____ Total possible points = _____ Points earned = _____

Evaluation Rubric Codes:
S = Satisfactory, meets standard   **U** = Unsatisfactory, fails to meet standard

Patient Preparation: Preanalytical Phase	Scores	
	S	**U**
1. Greeted the patient and confirmed identity while sanitizing hands..		
2. Explained procedure and how to disrobe (from the waist up with the gown opening in the front). Provided the patient with privacy.		
3. After returning, prepared the electrode sites by:		
a. Dry shaving hair (if necessary)		
b. Applying alcohol to remove lotions, oils, and dirt		
c. Rubbing the abrasive pad over the sites to increase circulation		
4. Noted the different configurations of where to place the **five** electrodes (and wires). Followed the manufacturer's diagram of the site locations or the physician's preference.		
5. Snapped the color-coded wires to their electrodes. One at a time, peeled the backing off of each sticky electrode with its colored lead wire and firmly pressed it on its appropriate prepared site. NOTE: Each Holter system provides its own diagram showing where each colored lead wire belongs.		
6. The wires coming from each electrode were looped and taped down with surgical tape or looped and held down by the lower sticky tab at the bottom of the electrode.		
7. Inserted the digital flashcard or tape into the Holter recorder. Placed the new batteries (provided in the supply kit) into the monitor, and connected the lead cable to the monitor.		

Procedure: Analytical Phase	Scores	
	S	U
8. Turned on the monitor and followed the manufacturer's directions for data input and quality control. Noted the start time on the monitor and wrote it in patient's log.		
9. Showed the patient the log book and how the monitor works and is stored in its pouch. Emphasized that the monitor and wires should not get wet.		
10. Instructed the patient to do the following in the log book (diary):		
- **Write down the activities** you do and exactly what time you do them using the clock on the Holter monitor screen. Activities include:		
- When you exert yourself		
- When you are at rest		
- When you eat		
- When you take medications		
- When you have bowel movements		
- **Write down any symptoms** you have while you are wearing the monitor, such as:		
- Chest pain		
- Shortness of breath		
- Lightheadedness		
- Skipped heartbeats		
- The physician will be comparing the data from the Holter monitor recorder with your diary, which will help diagnose your condition.		
11. Explained how long the patient will need to wear the monitor. (It may vary from 12 hours to 3 days or more based on the physician's order.)		
12. Documented in the patient record that all the above instructions were provided and when the patient was told to return.		

Follow-up: Postanalytical Phase	Scores	
	S	U
13. Performed the following when the monitoring period was over and the patient returned with the Holter monitor and the diary:		
- Checked to ensure entries were made in the log (diary).		
- Turned off and disconnected the monitor per manufacturer's instructions.		
- Disconnected the cable from the monitor.		
- Removed the monitor from the pouch.		
- Carefully removed electrodes from patient and the lead wires and discarded.		
- Cleaned the patient's chest of any residual gel from the electrodes.		
- Removed and discarded the batteries from the monitor.		
- Removed the flashcard/tape from the monitor and diary and turned it in for interpretation.		
- Cleaned Holter monitor and patient cable with lead wires for next patient		
14. Documented on patient chart (see below)		
15. Disinfected test area and instruments according to OSHA guidelines.		
Totals Counts per Column		

Patient Name: _____

Patient Chart Entry: (Include when, what, how, why, any additional information, and the signature of the person charting.)

_____

_____

10-4

Appendix: Forms for Documenting Safety, Quality Assurance, CLIA Compliance, Sample Health Assessment Form, and Professional Evaluation Form

CONTENTS

209

LABORATORY TECH RESPONSIBILITIES IN CLASSROOM LABORATORY

Full Name of Tech	Official Initials	Temp Check Date	Disinfected Counters	Other

211

Appendix: Forms for Documenting Safety, Quality Assurance

MONTHLY LABORATORY MAINTENANCE LOG

Medical Clinic							
Daily Maintenance Control Chart							
Month		**Year**					
	Daily					**Monthly**	
Day	**Refrig**	**Freezer**	**Room**	**Incubator**	**Bleach**	**Eye Wash**	**Shower**	**By**
	2-8° C	**−0-20° C**	**15-30° C**	**34-36° C**	**Counters**	**Checked**	**Checked**	
1								
2								
3								
4								
5								
6								
7								
8								
9								
10								
11								
12								
13								
14								
15								
16								
17								
18								
19								
20								
21								
22								
23								
24								
25								
26								
27								
28								
29								
30								
31								
Comments								

Exposure Event Number_____

Blood and Body Fluid Exposure Report Form

Facility name: _____

Name of exposed worker: Last: _____ **First:** _____ **ID#:** _____

Date of exposure: _____ / _____ / _____   **Time of exposure:** _____ : _____ **AM**   **PM** (Circle)

Job title/occupation: _____   **Department/work unit:** _____

Location where exposure occurred: _____

Name of person completing form: _____

Section I. Type of Exposure *(Check all that apply.)*

☐ **Percutaneous (Needle or sharp object that was in contact with blood or body fluids)**
(Complete Sections II, III, IV, and V.)

☐ **Mucocutaneous** *(Check below <u>and</u> complete Sections III, IV, and VI.)*
___ **Mucous Membrane**   ___ **Skin**

☐ **Bite** *(Complete Sections III, IV, and VI.)*

Section II. Needle/Sharp Device Information
(If exposure was <u>percutaneous</u>, provide the following information about the device involved.)

Name of device: _____   ☐ Unknown/Unable to determine

Brand/manufacturer: _____   ☐ Unknown/Unable to determine

Did the device have a sharps injury prevention feature, i.e., a "safety device"?

☐ Yes   ☐ No   ☐ Unknown/Unable to determine

If yes, when did the injury occur?

☐ Before activation of safety feature was appropriate   ☐ Safety feature failed after activation

☐ During activation of the safety feature   ☐ Safety feature not activated

☐ Safety feature improperly activated   ☐ Other: _____

Describe what happened with the safety feature, e.g., why it failed or why it was not activated: _____

_____

Section III. Employee Narrative *(Optional)*

Describe how the exposure occurred and how it might have been prevented:

_____

_____

_____

NOTE: <u>This is not a CDC or OSHA form.</u> This form was developed by CDC to help healthcare facilities with detailed exposure information that is specifically useful for the facilities' prevention planning. <u>Information on this page (#1)</u> <u>may</u> meet OSHA sharps injury documentation requirements and can be copied and filed for purposes of maintaining a separate sharps injury log. <u>Procedures for maintaining employee confidentiality must be followed.</u>

(Centers for Disease Control and Prevention,
http://www.cdc.gov/sharpssafety/pdf/AppendixA-7.doc)

213

Exposure Event Number_____

Section IV. Exposure and Source Information

A.   **Exposure Details:** *(Check all that apply.)*

     1.   **Type of fluid or material (For body fluid exposures <u>only</u>, check which fluid in adjacent box.)**

☐   Blood/blood products

☐   Visibly bloody body fluid*

☐   Non-visibly bloody body fluid*

☐   Visibly bloody solution (e.g., water used to clean a blood spill)

*Identify which body fluid		
___ Cerebrospinal	___ Urine	___ Synovial
___ Amniotic	___ Sputum	___ Peritoneal
___ Pericardial	___ Saliva	___ Semen/Vaginal
___ Pleural	___ Feces/stool	___ Other/Unknown

     2.   **Body site of exposure.** *(Check all that apply.)*

☐ Hand/finger   ☐ Eye   ☐ Mouth/nose   ☐ Face

☐ Arm   ☐ Leg   ☐ Other (Describe:_____)

     3.   **If percutaneous exposure:**

        Depth of injury *(Check only one.)*

☐   Superficial (e.g., scratch, no or little blood)

☐   Moderate (e.g., penetrated through skin, wound bled)

☐   Deep (e.g., intramuscular penetration)

☐   Unsure/Unknown

        Was blood visible on device before exposure?   ☐ Yes   ☐ No   ☐ Unsure/Unknown

     4.   **If mucous membrane or skin exposure:** *(Check only one.)*

        Approximate volume of material

☐   Small (e.g., few drops)

☐   Large (e.g., major blood splash)

        If skin exposure, was skin intact?   ☐ Yes   ☐ No   ☐ Unsure/Unknown

B.   **Source Information**

     1.   **Was the source individual identified?**   ☐ Yes   ☐ No   ☐ Unsure/Unknown

     2.   **Provide the serostatus of the source patient for the following pathogens.**

	Positive	**Negative**	**Refused**	**Unknown**
HIV Antibody	☐	☐	☐	☐
HCV Antibody	☐	☐	☐	☐
HbsAg	☐	☐	☐	☐

     3.   **If known, when was the serostatus of the source determined?**

☐   Known at the time of exposure

☐   Determined through testing at the time of or soon after the exposure

Section V. Percutaneous Injury Circumstances

A. **What device or item caused the injury?**

Hollow-bore needle

☐ Hypodermic needle

__ Attached to syringe __ Attached to IV tubing __ Unattached

☐ Prefilled cartridge syringe needle

☐ Winged steel needle (i.e., butterfly type devices)

__ Attached to syringe, tube holder, or IV tubing __ Unattached

☐ IV stylet

☐ Phlebotomy needle

☐ Spinal or epidural needle

☐ Bone marrow needle

☐ Biopsy needle

☐ Huber needle

☐ Other type of hollow-bore needle (type: _____)

☐ Hollow-bore needle, type unknown

Suture needle

☐ Suture needle

Glass

☐ Capillary tube

☐ Pipette (glass)

☐ Slide

☐ Specimen/test/vacuum

☐ Other: _____

Other sharp objects

☐ Bone chip/chipped tooth

☐ Bone cutter

☐ Bovie electrocautery device

☐ Bur

☐ Explorer

☐ Extraction forceps

☐ Elevator

☐ Histology cutting blade

☐ Lancet

☐ Pin

☐ Razor

☐ Retractor

☐ Rod (orthopaedic applications)

☐ Root canal file

☐ Scaler/curette

☐ Scalpel blade

☐ Scissors

☐ Tenaculum

☐ Trocar

☐ Wire

☐ Other type of sharp object

☐ Sharp object, type unknown

Other device or item

☐ Other: _____

B. **Purpose or procedure for which sharp item was used or intended.**
(Check one procedure type and complete information in corresponding box as applicable.)

☐ Establish intravenous or arterial access (Indicate type of line.)————→

☐ Access established intravenous or arterial line (Indicate type of line and reason for line access.)———

☐ Injection through skin or mucous membrane (Indicate type of injection.)—

☐ Obtain blood specimen (through skin) (Indicate method of specimen collection.)

☐ Other specimen collection

☐ Suturing

☐ Cutting

☐ Other procedure

☐ Unknown

Type of Line

__ Peripheral   __ Arterial
__ Central   __ Other

Reason for Access

__ Connect IV infusion/piggyback
__ Flush with heparin/saline
__ Obtain blood specimen
__ Inject medication
__ Other: _____

Type of Injection

__ IM injection   __ Epidural/spinal anesthesia
__ Skin test placement   __ Other injection
__ Other ID/SQ injection

Type of Blood Sampling

__ Venipuncture   __ Umbilical vessel
__ Arterial puncture   __ Finger/heelstick
__ Dialysis/AV fistula site   __ Other blood sampling

Appendix: Forms for Documenting Safety, Quality Assurance

C. **When and how did the injury occur? (From the left hand side of page, select the point during or after use that most closely represents when the injury occurred. In the corresponding right-hand box, select *one* or *two* circumstances that reflect how the injury happened.)**

☐ During use of the item ⟶

Select one or two choices:

___ Patient moved and jarred device
___ While inserting needle/sharp
___ While manipulating needle/sharp
___ While withdrawing needle/sharp
___ Passing or receiving equipment
___ Suturing
___ Tying sutures
___ Manipulating suture needle in holder
___ Incising
___ Palpating/exploring
___ Collided with co-worker or other during procedure
___ Collided with sharp during procedure
___ Sharp object dropped during procedure

☐ After use, before disposal of item ⟶

Select one or two choices:

___ Handling equipment on a tray or stand
___ Transferring specimen into specimen container
___ Processing specimens
___ Passing or transferring equipment
___ Recapping (missed or pierced cap)
___ Cap fell off after recapping
___ Disassembling device or equipment
___ Decontamination/processing of used equipment
___ During clean-up
___ In transit to disposal
___ Opening/breaking glass containers
___ Collided with co-worker/other person
___ Collided with sharp after procedure
___ Sharp object dropped after procedure
___ Struck by detached IV line needle

☐ During or after disposal of item ⟶

☐ Other (Describe): _____

_____

_____

_____

☐ Unknown

Select one or two choices:

___ Placing sharp in container:
  ___ Injured by sharp being disposed
  ___ Injured by sharp already in container
___ While manipulating container
___ Over-filled sharps container
___ Punctured sharps container
___ Sharp protruding from open container
___ Sharp in unusual location:
  ___ In trash
  ___ In linen/laundry
  ___ Left on table/tray
  ___ Left in bed/mattress
  ___ On floor
  ___ In pocket/clothing
  ___ Other unusual location
___ Collided with co-worker or other person
___ Collided with sharp
___ Sharp object dropped
___ Struck by detached IV line needle

Section VI. Mucous Membrane Exposures Circumstances

A. **What barriers were used by worker at the time of the exposure?** *(Check all that apply.)*

☐ Gloves   ☐ Goggles   ☐ Eyeglasses   ☐ Face Shield   ☐ Mask   ☐ Gown

B. **Activity/Event when exposure occurred** *(Check one.)*

☐ Patient spit/coughed/vomited
☐ Airway manipulation (e.g., suctioning airway, inducing sputum)
☐ Endoscopic procedure
☐ Dental procedure
☐ Tube placement/removal/manipulation (e.g., chest, endotracheal, NG, rectal, urine catheter)
☐ Phlebotomy
☐ IV or arterial line insertion/removal/manipulation
☐ Irrigation procedure
☐ Vaginal delivery
☐ Surgical procedure (e.g., all surgical procedures including C-section)
☐ Bleeding vessel
☐ Changing dressing/wound care
☐ Manipulating blood tube/bottle/specimen container
☐ Cleaning/transporting contaminated equipment
☐ Other: _____
☐ Unknown

Comments: _____

_____

_____

_____

_____

_____

_____

_____

_____

217

GENERIC QUALITATIVE CONTROL AND PATIENT LOG (TEMPLATE)

Test: _____

Kit Name and Manufacturer: _____

Lot #: _____   Expiration Date: _____

Storage Requirements: _____   Test Flow Chart: _____

Date	Tech Initials	Specimen ID (Control/Patient)	Result (+ or −)	Internal Control Passed (Y or N)	Charted in Patient Record

Appendix: Forms for Documenting Safety, Quality Assurance

GENERIC QUANTITATIVE TEST CONTROL LOG (TEMPLATE)

Control Lot #: _____   Expiration Date: _____

Control Range: _____   Control Level: _____

Date	Tech	Result	Accept	Reject	Corrective Action

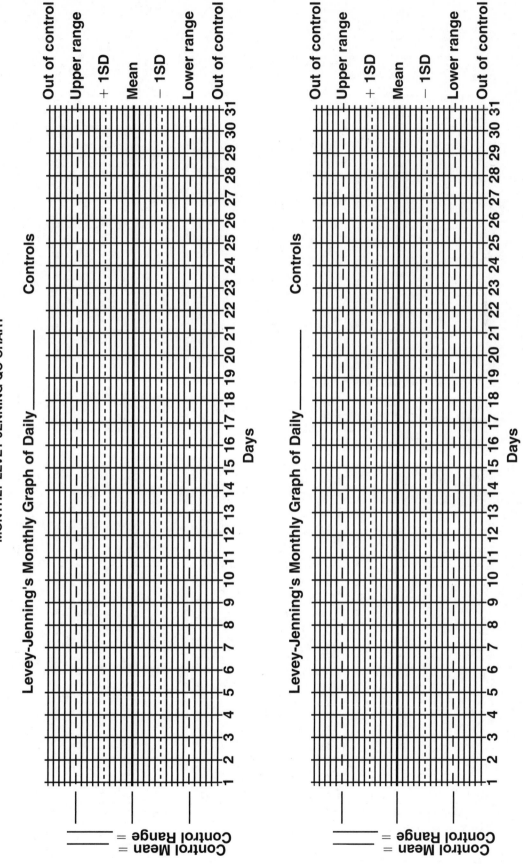

MONTHLY LEVEY-JENNING QC CHART

Appendix: Forms for Documenting Safety, Quality Assurance

URINE DIPSTICK QUALITY CONTROL LOG

DATE_____ URINE DIPSTICK CONTROL LEVEL _____ LOT #_____ EXPIRATION DATE_____

DATE	Reagent Strip / Lot # / Patient	DIPSTICK TESTS										CONFIRMATORY TESTS								ADD. TESTS		INITIAL
		Leukocytes	Nitrites	Urobilinogen	Protein	pH	Blood	Specific Gravity	Ketones	Bilirubin	Glucose	Protein	Method/Lot #	Ketones	Method/Lot #	Glucose	Method/Lot #	Bilirubin	Method/Lot #	hCG	Method/Lot #	Specific Gravity Refractometer

Appendix: Forms for Documenting Safety, Quality Assurance

URINE DIPSTICK PATIENT LOG

DATE	Reagent Strip Lot# Patient	Leukocytes	Nitrites	Urobilinogen	Protein	pH	Blood	Specific Gravity	Ketones	Bilirubin	Glucose	Protein	Method/Lot #	Ketones	Method/Lot #	Glucose	Method/Lot #	Bilirubin	Method/Lot #	hCG	Method/Lot #	Specific Gravity Refractometer	INITIAL
								DIPSTICK TESTS					CONFIRMATORY TESTS							ADD. TESTS			

Sample Device Preselection Worksheet

Type of Device: _____ Name: _____ Manufacturer: _____

Clinical Considerations	Does this consideration apply to this device?		If Yes, what is the level of importance?		
	No	Yes	High	Med	Low
Device use will require a change in technique (compared to conventional product).					
Device permits needle changes.					
Device permits reuse of the needle on the same patient during a procedure. (e.g., local anesthesia)					
Device allows easy visualization of flashback.					
Device allows easy visualization of medication.					
Other:					
Comment:					

Procedural Implications for Healthcare Provider

Clinical Considerations		Does this consideration apply to this device?		If Yes, what is the level of importance?		
		No	Yes	High	Med	Low
Patient Considerations	Device is latex free.					
	Device has potential for causing infection.					
	Device has potential for causing increased pain or discomfort to patients.					
	Other:					
	Comment:					
Scope of Device Use Considerations	Device can be used with adult and pediatric populations.					
	Specialty areas (e.g., OR, anesthesiology, radiology) can use the device.					
	Device can be used for all same purposes for which the conventional device is used.					
	Device is available in all currently used sizes.					
	Other:					
	Comment:					

226

Safety Considerations	Does this consideration apply to this device?		If Yes, what is the level of importance?		
	No	Yes	High	Med	Low
Method Activation					
The safety feature does not require activation by the user.					
The worker's hands can remain behind the sharp during activation of the safety.					
Activation of the safety feature can be performed with one hand.					
Other:					
Comment:					
Characteristics of the Safety Feature					
The safety feature is in effect during use in the patient.					
The safety feature permanently isolates the sharp.					
The safety feature is integrated into the device (i.e., does not need to be added before use).					
A visible or audible cue provides evidence of safety feature activation.					
The safety feature is easy to recognize and intuitive to use.					
Other:					
Comment:					

Appendix: Forms for Documenting Safety, Quality Assurance

Other Considerations

	Other Considerations	Does this consideration apply to this device?		If Yes, what is the level of importance?		
		No	Yes	High	Med	Low
Availability	The device is available in all sizes currently used in the organization.					
	The manufacturer can provide the device in needed quantities.					
Service Provided	The company representative will assist with training.					
	Product materials are available to assist with training.					
	The company will provide free samples for evaluation.					
	The company has a history of being responsive when problems arise.					
	Comment:					
Practical Considerations	The device will **not** increase the volume of sharps waste.					
	The device will **not** require changes in the size or shape of sharps containers.					
	Other:					
	Comment:					

Centers for Disease Control and Prevention, "Sample Device Pre-Selection Worksheet," Sharps Injury Prevention Workbook, A-12, http://www.cdc.gov/sharpssafety/index.html.

SAMPLE DEVICE EVALUATION FORM

Product: _____   Date: _____

Department/unit: _____   Position/title: _____

1. **Number of times you used the device.**

   ☐ 1–5   ☐ 6–10   ☐ 11–25   ☐ 26–50   ☐ More than 50

2. **Please mark the box that best describes your experiences with the device. If a question is not applicable to this device, do not fill in an answer for that question.**

Factors	Strongly Disagree	Disagree	Neither Agree nor Disagree	Agree	Strongly Agree
Patient/Procedure Considerations					
a. Needle penetration **is** comparable to the standard device.	1	2	3	4	5
b. Patients/residents **do not** perceive more pain or discomfort with this device.	1	2	3	4	5
c. Use of the device **does not** increase the number of repeat sticks of patient.	1	2	3	4	5
d. The device **does not** increase the time it takes to perform the procedure.	1	2	3	4	5
e. Use of the device **does not** require a change in procedural technique.	1	2	3	4	5
f. The device is compatible with other equipment that must be used with it.	1	2	3	4	5
g. The device can be used for the same purposes as the standard device.	1	2	3	4	5
h. Use of the device **is not** affected by my hand size.	1	2	3	4	5
i. Age or size of patient/resident **does not** affect use of this device.	1	2	3	4	5
Experience with the Safety Feature					
j. Safety feature **does not** interfere with procedural technique.	1	2	3	4	5
k. The safety feature is easy to activate.	1	2	3	4	5
l. Safety feature **does not** activate before the procedure is completed.	1	2	3	4	5
m. Once activated, the safety feature remains engaged.	1	2	3	4	5
n. I **did not** experience any injury or *near miss* of injury with the device.	1	2	3	4	5

Appendix: Forms for Documenting Safety, Quality Assurance

Special Questions about This Device					
[To be added by health care facility]	1	2	3	4	5
	1	2	3	4	5
	1	2	3	4	5
Overall Rating					
Overall, the device is effective for patient and resident care and safety.	1	2	3	4	5

3. Did you participate in training on how to use this product?

☐ No *(Go to question 6.)*   ☐ Yes *(Go to next question.)*

4. Who provided this instruction? *(Check all that apply.)*

☐ Product representative   ☐ Staff development personnel   ☐ Other _____

5. Was the training you received adequate?

☐ No   ☐ Yes

6. Was special training needed to use the product effectively?

☐ No   ☐ Yes

7. Compared with others of your gender, how would you describe your hand size?

☐ Small   ☐ Medium   ☐ Large

8. What is your gender?

☐ Female   ☐ Male

9. Which of the following do you consider yourself to be?

☐ Left-handed   ☐ Right-handed

10. Please add any additional comments below.

_____

_____

THANK YOU FOR COMPLETING THIS SURVEY

Please return this form to _____

(Centers for Disease Control and Prevention, Sample Device Evaluation Form, Sharps Injury Prevention Workbook, A-13; http://www.cdc.gov/sharpssafety/index.html)

LABORATORY REQUISITION
Biomedical Laboratories, Inc.
100 Main Street
Athens, Georgia 45760

☐ Fax   Send additional copy of report to:

☐ Call   Client Number/Physician's Name   Phone/Fax number ( )

☐ Mail   Physician's Address   City, State, Zip

Patient's Name (Last)	(First)	(MI)	Sex	Date of Birth MO | DAY | YEAR	Collection Time : AM PM	Fasting YES NO	Collection Date MO | DAY | YEAR

NPI/UPIN	Physician's ID #	Patient's SS #	Patient's ID #	Urine hrs/vol hrs_____ vol ____

PATIENT

Physician's Name (Last, First)	Physician's Signature	Patient's Address	Phone
Medicare # (Include prefix/suffix)	☐ Primary ☐ Secondary	City	State ZIP
Medicaid # State	Physician's Provider #	Name of Responsible Party (if different from patient)	

RESP. PARTY

Diagnosis/Signs/Symptoms in ICD-9 Format (Highest Specificity)	Address of Responsible Party (if different from patient) APT #

REQUIRED

City   State   ZIP

INSURANCE

Patient's Relationship to Responsible Party   ☐ 1–Self   ☐ 2–Spouse   ☐ 3–Child   ☐ 4–Other

Performance Lab ☐	Carrier	Group #	Employee #	Mem

Insurance Company Name	Plan	Carrier Code
Subscriber/Member #	Location	Group #
Insurance Address	Physician's Provider #	
City	State	ZIP
Employer's Name or Number	Insured SS # (If not patient)	Worker's Comp ☐ Yes ☐ No

I hereby authorize the release of medical information related to the service subscribed herein and authorize payment directed to LabCorp.

X _____ _____
Patient's Signature   Date

MEDICARE ADVANCE BENEFICIARY NOTICE

I have read the ABN on the reverse. If Medicare denies payment, I agree to pay for the identified test(s).

X _____ _____
Patient's Signature   Date

NOTE: WHEN ORDERING TESTS FOR WHICH MEDICARE OR MEDICAID REIMBURSEMENT WILL BE SOUGHT, PHYSICIANS SHOULD ONLY ORDER TESTS THAT ARE MEDICALLY NECESSARY FOR THE DIAGNOSIS OR TREATMENT OF THE PATIENT. COMPONENTS OF THE ORGAN OR DISEASE PANELS/COMBINATIONS PRINTED BELOW ARE SHOWN ON THE REVERSE SIDE AND MAY ALSO BE ORDERED INDIVIDUALLY BELOW. COMPONENTS MAY BE BILLED SEPARATELY PER CARRIER POLICY.

PROFILES (See reverse for components)

Code	Test	Tube
80049	Basic Metabolic Profile	SST
80054	Comp Metabolic Profile	SST
80051	Electrolyte Profile	SST
80058	Hepatic Profile	SST
80059	Hepatitis Profile	SST
80061	Lipid Profile	SST
80091	Thyroid Profile	SST
80055	Prenatal Profile	RED LAV
80072	Rheumatoid Profile	SST

HEMATOLOGY/COAGULATION

Code	Test	Tube
85025	CBC w Diff	LAV
85027	CBC w/o Diff	LAV
85014	Hematocrit	LAV
85018	Hemoglobin	LAV
85595	Platelet Count	LAV
85041	RBC Count	LAV
85048	WBC Count	LAV
85007	WBC Differential	LAV
89190	Nasal Smear, Eosin	Nasal Smear
85060	Pathologist Consult–Peripheral Smear	LAV
85651	Sed Rate	LAV
85610	Prothrombin Time (PT)	BLU
86900 86901	PT and PTT Activated	BLU
85730	PTT Activated	BLU

CHEMISTRY

Code	Test	Tube
82040	Albumin	SST
84075	Alkaline Phosphatase	SST
84460	ALT (SGPT)	SST
82150	Amylase, Serum	SST
84450	AST (SGOT)	SST

ALPHABETICAL TESTS CON'T

Code	Test	Tube
82607 82746	B₁₂ and Folate	SST
82250	Bilirubin, Total	SST
84520	BUN	SST
82310	Calcium	SST
82378	CEA	SST
82465	Cholesterol, Total	SST
82565	Creatinine	SST
82670	Estradiol	SST
82728	Ferritin, Serum	SST
82985	Fructosamine	SST
83001	FSH	SST
83001 83002	FSH and LH	SST
82977	GGT	SST
82947	Glucose, Plasma	GRY
82947	Glucose, Serum	SST
82950	Glucose, 2-hr. PP	SST
83036	Glycohemoglobin, Total	LAV
84703	hCG, Beta Subunit, Qual	SST
84702	hCG, Beta Subunit, Quant	SST
83718	HDL Cholesterol	SST
83036	Hemoglobin A₁C	LAV

SEROLOGY/IMMUNOLOGY

Code	Test	Tube
85610 85730	ABO and Rh	LAV
86038	Antinuclear Antibodies	SST
86677	Helicobacter pylori, IgG	SST
86706	Hep B Surface Antibody	SST
87340	Hep B Surface Antigen	SST
86803	Hep C Antibody	SST
86701	HIV Antibodies Serology	SST

ALPHABETICAL TESTS CON'T

Code	Test	Tube
83540	Iron, Total	SST
83540 83550	Iron and IBC	SST
83615	LDH	SST
83002	LH	SST
83690	Lipase	SER
83735	Magnesium, Serum	SST
84132	Potassium	SST
84146	Prolactin, Serum	SST
84153	Prostate-Specific Antigen	SST
84066	Prostatic Acid Phos	SST
84155	Protein, Total	SST
86431	Rheumatoid Arthritis Factor	SST
86592	RPR	SST
86762	Rubella Antibodies, IgG	SST
84295	Sodium	SST
84403	Testosterone	SST
84436	Thyroxine (T₄)	SST
84478	Triglycerides	SST
84480	Triiodothyronine (T₃)	SST
84443	TSH, High Sensitivity	SST
84550	Uric Acid	SST

TOXICOLOGY

Code	Test	Tube
80156	Carbamazepine (Tegretol®)	SER
80162	Digoxin	SER
80178	Lithium (Eskalith®)	SER
80184	Phenobarbital (Luminal®)	SER
80185	Phenytoin (Dilantin®)	SER
80198	Theophylline Toxicology	SER
80164	Valproic Acid (Depakene®)	SER

URINALYSIS

Code	Test		Tube
81003	Urinalysis	Microscopic on Positives	URN
81001	Urinalysis	with Microscopic	URN

MICROBIOLOGY   See Reverse Side

☐ ENDOCERVICAL   ☐ THROAT   ☐ URINE
☐ STOOL   ☐ URETHRAL   INDICATE SOURCE

Code	Test	Tube
87070	Aerobic Bacterial Culture	Bact Trnspt
87490 87590	Chlamydia/GC DNA Probe w/ Confirmation on Positives	Probe Trnspt
87490 87590	Chlamydia/GC DNA Probe Without Confirmation	Probe Trnspt
87490	Chlamydia DNA Probe	Probe Trnspt
87081	Genital, Beta-Hemolytic Strep Cult, Group B	Bact Trnspt
87070	Genital Culture, Routine	Bact Trnspt
87070	Lower Respiratory Culture	Steril Trnspt
87590	N. gonorrhoeae DNA Probe	Probe Trnspt
87015 87211	Ova and Parasites	O & P Kit
87081 X2 87045	Stool Culture	Fecal Trnspt
87081	Throat, Beta-Hemolytic Strep Cult, Group A	Bact Trnspt
87060	Upper Respiratory Culture, Routine	Bact Trnspt
87086	Urine Culture, Routine	Urn Cul Trnspt

Clinical Information/Comments

OTHER TESTS/INDIVIDUAL COMPONENTS

TEST #   TEST NAMES

LAB USE ONLY	STAT ☐ 998074	VENIPUNCTURE ☐ 998085	TRAVEL ☐ 998096	NON LABCORP ☐ 998239	VERBAL ORDER ☐ 998250	CHART ORDER ☐ 998261	HANDWRITTEN ☐ 998272	24 HR TUV ☐ 998283	PST/PSC #

CONTAINERS RECEIVED → | SST SPUN | USST UNSPUN | SER SERUM | FRZ FRZ TRNS | RED RED | LAV LAVENDER | SLD SLIDE | BLU LT. BLUE | GRY GREY | GRN GREEN | RYB RYL BLU | YEL ACD | PLS PLASMA | URN URINE | 24U 24 HR URINE | TA-U TART. ACID | FL FLUID | OT OTHER | BACT TRNSP | O & P KIT | PROBE TRNSP | URN CUL TRNSP | STERIL TRNSP | FECAL TRNSP | VIRAL TRNSP |

300-0384

231

SPECIMEN LOG SHEET

Date Sent	Tech Initials	PT. #	Doctor	Tests Ordered	Tubes Sent	Lab to Pick Up	Results Received

Quality Control Flow Chart for HemoCue

Regardless of the purpose, most clinical testing procedures have the same quality control requirements. If an instrument is used, there is usually a method to check its mechanical function. Often this is nothing more than an "optic check" or calibration strip supplied with the instrument to allow the user to determine whether the instrument is functional.

After determining that the instrument does indeed function, one then needs to prove that the reagents will perform as expected. Commonly, one uses a high and low value control sample. Look at the results. Are they within their expected ranges? If so, you can begin to test patients. If not, then it is time to do some troubleshooting.

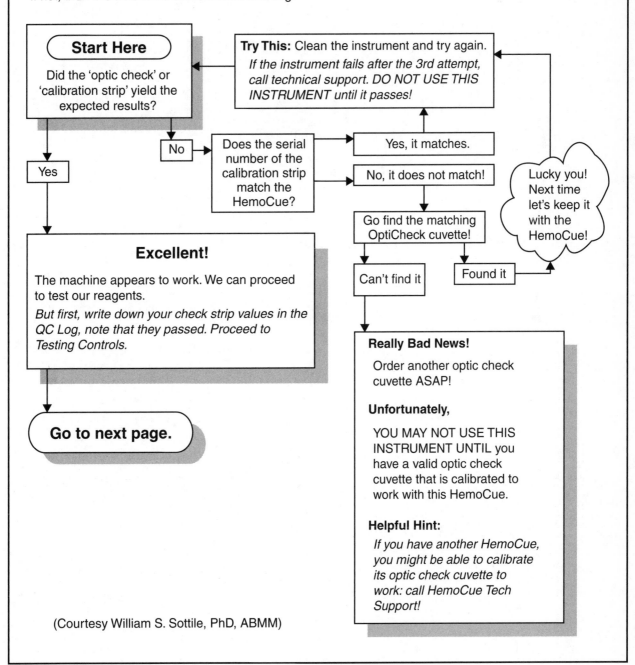

(Courtesy William S. Sottile, PhD, ABMM)

HEMOGLOBIN QUALITY CONTROL LOG

Test: _____   Control Lot #: _____

Control Range: _____   For Low/Normal/High Control

Date	Tech	Result	Accept	Reject	Corrective Action

Appendix: Forms for Documenting Safety, Quality Assurance

HEMOGLOBIN PATIENT LOG

Test: _____   Kit Lot #: _____

Expected Hemoglobin Values:

Adult males = 13.0–18 g/dL   Adult females = 11.0–16.0 g/dL

Infants = 10.0–14.0 g/dL   Children = Increase to adult

Date	Tech	Patient ID	Result	Charted

Appendix: Forms for Documenting Safety, Quality Assurance

HEMATOCRIT QUALITY CONTROL LOG

Test: _____   Control Lot #: _____

Control Range : _____   For Low/Normal/High Control

Date	Tech	Slot #	Result	Accept	Reject	Corrective Action

Appendix: Forms for Documenting Safety, Quality Assurance

HEMATOCRIT PATIENT LOG

Expected Hematocrit Values:

Adult males = 42–52%   Adult females = 36–48%

Infants = 32–38%   Children = Increase to adult

Date	Tech	Patient ID	Slot #	Result	Charted

ERYTHROCYTE SEDIMENTATION RATE PATIENT LOG

Expected ESR Values:

Adult males < 50 yr = 0–15 mm/hr   Adult females < 50 yr = 0–20 mm/hr

Adult males > 50 yr = 0–20 mm/hr   Adult females > 50 yr = 0–30 mm/hr

Date	Tech	Patient ID	Slot #	Time	Result	Charted

Appendix: Forms for Documenting Safety, Quality Assurance

PROTIME PATIENT LOG

ProTime expected values for normal and therapeutic whole blood:

	INR	PT (seconds; see ranges in insert)
Normal	0.8–1.2	_____
Low anticoagulation	1.5–2.0	_____
Moderate anticoagulation	2.0–3.0	_____
High anticoagulation	2.5–4.0	_____

Date	Tech	Patient ID	INR	PT (seconds)	Charted

GENERIC QUANTITATIVE TEST PROCEDURE (TEMPLATE)

Quantitative Test _____

Person evaluated _____   **Date** _____

Evaluated by _____   **Score/Grade** _____

Outcome goal:	
Conditions:	
Standards:	Required time = _____ minutes Performance time = _____ Total possible points = _____ Points earned = _____

Evaluation Rubric Codes:
S = Satisfactory—Meets standard   **U** = Unsatisfactory—Fails to meet standard

NOTE: Steps marked with an asterisk (*) are critical to achieve required competency.

Preparation: Preanalytical Phase	Scores	
	S	U
A. Test information		
- Kit or instrumental method: _____		
- Manufacturer: _____		
- Proper storage (e.g., temperature, light): _____		
- Lot number of kit or supplies: _____		
- Expiration date: _____		
- Package insert and/or test flow chart available: yes _____ no _____		
B. Specimen information		
- Type of specimen and its preparation (e.g., fasting, first morning): _____		
- Specimen container or testing device: _____		
- Amount of specimen: _____		
C. Personal protective equipment (PPE): _____		
D. Assembled all the above, sanitized hands, and applied PPE.		

Procedure: Analytical Phase	Scores	
	S	U
E. Performed/observed quality control for A or B below.		
Quantitative testing controls		
- Calibration check: _____		
- Control levels: Normal _____ High _____ Low _____		

241

F. Performed patient test: Followed proper steps (see flow chart and list steps).	S	U
1.		
2.		
3.		
4.		
5.		
6.		
7.		
8.		
9.		
10.		

*Accurate Results _____   Instructor Confirmation _____

Follow-up: Postanalytical	Scores	
	S	U
*G. Proper documentation		
1. On control log _____ yes _____ no		
2. On patient log _____ yes _____ no		
3. Documentation on patient chart (see below)		
4. Identified "critical values" and took appropriate steps to notify physician.		
EXPECTED VALUES FOR ANALYTE:		
H. Proper disposal and disinfection		
1. Disposed of all sharps into biohazard sharps containers.		
2. Disposed of all other regulated medical waste into biohazard bags.		
3. Disinfected test area and instruments according to OSHA guidelines.		
4. Sanitized hands after removing gloves.		
Column Totals		

Patient Name: _____

Patient Chart Entry: (Include when, what, how, why, any additional information, and the signature of the person charting.)

_____

_____

_____

Appendix: Forms for Documenting Safety, Quality Assurance

GLUCOSE TEST CONTROL LOG

Control Lot #: _____   Expiration Date: _____

Control Range: _____   Level: Low/Normal/High

Date	Tech	Result	Accept	Reject	Corrective Action

Appendix: Forms for Documenting Safety, Quality Assurance

GLUCOSE PATIENT LOG

Date	Tech	Patient	Result	Charted

HEMOGLOBIN A$_{1c}$ PATIENT/CONTROL LOG

Date	Tech	Patient	Result	Charted

Appendix: Forms for Documenting Safety, Quality Assurance

CHOLESTECH LDX PATIENT/CONTROL LOG

Cassette Lot #: _____   Expiration Date: _____   LDX Serial #: _____

Date	Operator	Patient ID	Charted	TRG	TC	GLU	HDL	LDL	TC/ HDL	ALT

246

HEMOCCULT PATIENT LOG

Date	Tech	Patient	Result

Appendix: Forms for Documenting Safety, Quality Assurance

I-STAT PATIENT/CONTROL LOG

Cartridge Lot #: _____

Expiration Date: _____

Serial #: _____

Date	Operator	Patient ID	Charted	Na	K	Cl	TCO₂	iCa	Glu	BUN	Crea	Hct	Hb	AnGap

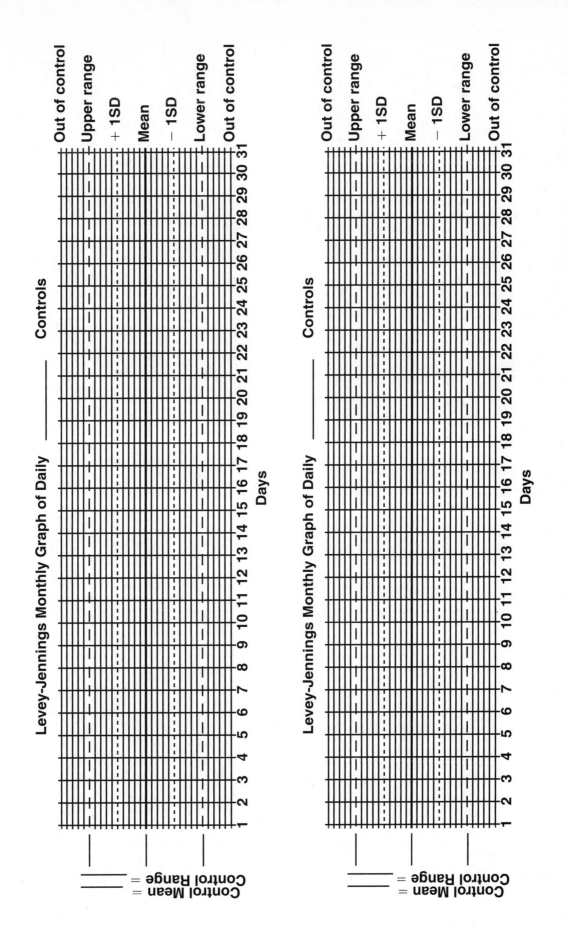

Appendix: Forms for Documenting Safety, Quality Assurance

QUALITATIVE CONTROL AND PATIENT LOG FOR IMMUNOLOGY
AND MICROBIOLOGY TEST KITS (TEMPLATE)

Test: _____

Kit Name and Manufacturer: _____

Lot # _____   **Expiration Date:** _____

Storage Requirements: _____   **Test Flow Chart:** _____

Date	Tech Initials	Specimen ID (Control/Patient)	Result (+ or −)	Internal Control Passed (Y or N)	Charted in Patient Record

Appendix: Forms for Documenting Safety, Quality Assurance

GENERIC QUALITATIVE TEST PROCEDURE (TEMPLATE)

Qualitative Test _____

Person evaluated _____ **Date** _____

Evaluated by _____ **Score/Grade** _____

Outcome goal:	
Conditions:	Supplies required:
Standards:	Required time = _____ minutes Performance time = _____ Total possible points = _____ Points earned = _____

Evaluation Rubric Codes:
S = Satisfactory—Meets standard   **U** = Unsatisfactory—Fails to meet standard

NOTE: Steps marked with an asterisk (*) are critical to achieve required competency.

Preparation: Preanalytical Phase	Scores	
	S	U
A. Test information		
- Kit method:		
- Manufacturer:		
- Proper storage (e.g., temperature, light):		
- Lot number of kit: _____		
- Expiration date: _____		
- Package insert and/or test flow chart available: _____ yes _____ no		
B. Personal protective equipment		
C. Specimen information		

Procedure: Analytical Phase	Scores	
	S	U
D. Performed/observed qualitative quality control		
- External liquid controls: Positive _____ Negative _____		
- Internal control:		
E. Performed patient test	**S**	**U**
1.		
2.		
3.		
4.		

POSITIVE seen as:

NEGATIVE seen as:

INVALID seen as:

*Accurate Results _____   **Instructor Confirmation** _____

Follow-up: Postanalytical Phase	Scores	
	S	**U**
*F. Proper documentation		
1. On control/patient log: _____ yes _____ no		
2. Documentation on patient chart (see below)		
3. Identified "critical values" and took appropriate steps to notify physician. EXPECTED VALUES FOR ANALYTE:		
G. Proper disposal and disinfection		
1. Disposed of all sharps into biohazard sharps containers.		
2. Disposed of all other regulated medical waste into biohazard bags.		
3. Disinfected test area and instruments according to OSHA guidelines.		
4. Sanitized hands after removing gloves.		
Column Totals		

Patient Name: _____

Patient Chart Entry: (Include when, what, how, why, any additional information, and the signature of the person charting.)

_____

_____

_____

Appendix: Forms for Documenting Safety, Quality Assurance

SAMPLE HEALTH ASSESSMENT FORM

Please print clearly: Date _____

Name _____   Address _____

City _____   State _____   ZIP _____

Telephone _____   Age (date of birth) ____/ ____/ ____

Sex _____   Race _____   Ht. _____   Wt. _____

Do you consider yourself overweight? _____   If so, how much? _____

Name of family doctor _____   When last seen? _____

Do you smoke? _____   If yes, how many packs per day _____   Alcohol use? _____

Do you have   _____ Heart trouble   _____ High blood pressure

                              _____ Kidney problems   _____ Heart attack before/after 40

Are you taking medication for cholesterol? _____   Blood pressure? _____   Other? _____

Do you exercise regularly? _____   When did you last eat? _____ hours

---

When you are finished with all your tests, please return to this room for final review of your results.

RELEASE:

I RELEASE _____ and the Health Technology Students from any liability as a result of my participation in this free Health Fair.

Signature _____   Date _____

Parent/Guardian _____   Witness _____

Appendix: Forms for Documenting Safety, Quality Assurance

TEST	NORMAL LIMITS	RESULTS	FURTHER EVALUATION _____

URINALYSIS ☐

Glucose	NEG	
Bilirubin	NEG	
Ketone	NEG	
Spec grav	1.005–1.030	
Blood	NEG	
pH	6.0–8.0	
Protein	NEG/TRACE	
Urobil.	NORM	
Nitrite	NEG	
Leukocytes	NEG	

Clinitek: asterisk (*) indicates further evaluation

Urinalysis
Routine urinalysis is a basic test, but it provides the physician with a tremendous amount of information about a disease. This test can help confirm or rule out a suspected diagnosis. It is a routine test that is repeated annually or as frequently as necessary to evaluate the patient's health status.

HEMATOLOGY

Anemia   Hemoglobin: >12 gm or g/dL   _____   ☐

Hematocrit: >32%   _____   ☐

Anemia Check
The hemoglobin and hematocrit tests determine the oxygen-carrying ability of the blood. They are simple and efficient methods to detect any anemia. A patient is considered anemic if the hemoglobin value is < 12 mg/dL or the hematocrit is < 34%. Low values are caused by hemorrhage, pregnancy, recent menstruation, iron deficiency, or other conditions that the physician needs to evaluate.

Erythrocyte Sedimentation Rate (ESR) = 0–20 mm/hr _____   ☐
Erythrocyte sedimentation rates are increased in infectious and inflammatory diseases, tissue destruction, and other conditions that increase the plasma fibrinogen level.

COAGULATION

INRatio   _____ INR

ProTime   _____ seconds

> Desirable <u>0.8–1.2</u> INR
>
> Therapeutic <u>1.5–4.0</u> INR
>
> PT = _____ seconds

BLOOD CHEMISTRY

Glucose

    Fasting _____ (8 or more hours since eating)

    Random (hours since eating) _____ hr

    Normal 80–125 (if 2 hr after eating) _____

Hemoglobin A$_{1c}$ **Desirable levels are < 7%**   **Result** _____

WARNING SIGNS OF DIABETES	
Type 1 Diabetes	**Type 2 Diabetes**
Constant urination Abnormal thirst Unusual hunger Rapid loss of weight Irritability Obvious weakness or fatigue Nausea and vomiting	Drowsiness Itching A family history of diabetes Blurred vision Excessive weight Tingling, numbness in feet Easy fatigue Skin infections and slow healing

LIPID PROFILE (CHOLESTECH TEST)

Lipid Profile	Desirable Numbers	Cholestech Results
Total cholesterol	< 200 mg/dL	
HDL cholesterol	> 40 mg/dL	
LDL cholesterol	< 130 mg/dL	
Triglycerides	< 150 mg/dL	
TC/HDL ratio	4.5 or less	
Glucose	Fasting: 60-110 mg/dL	
	Nonfasting: < 160 mg/dL	

Cholesterol

Cholesterol measurements are used to diagnose and monitor disorders involving excess cholesterol in the blood and fat metabolism disorders. These conditions often are associated with coronary heart disease. It is thought that lowering mean cholesterol levels can reduce coronary heart disease.

    Appendix: Forms for Documenting Safety, Quality Assurance

CHEMISTRY PROFILE I-STAT (Chem 8+)

Test	Test Symbol	Units	Reference Range	Result
Sodium	Na	mmol/L	138–146	
Potassium	K	mmol/L	3.5–4.9	
Chloride	Cl	mmol/L	98–109	
Total carbon dioxide	TCO_2	mmol/L	24–29	
Ionized calcium	iCa	mmol/L	1.12–1.32	
Glucose	Glu	mg/dL	70–105	
Urea nitrogen	BUN	mg/dL	8–26	
Creatinine	Crea	mg/dL	0.6–1.3	
Hematocrit	Hct	% PCV	38–51	
Hemoglobin*	Hb	g/dL	12–17	
Anion gap*	AnGap	mmol/L	10–20	

* These results are figured mathematically from the other results (not directly).

FECAL OCCULT BLOOD

Results: Positive _____ Negative _____

ECG AND SPIROMETRY: See attached reports.

REVIEW OF ALL RESULTS:

Appendix: Forms for Documenting Safety, Quality Assurance

PROFESSIONAL EVALUATION FORM FOR THE LABORATORY CLASSROOM

Student: _____ **Date:** _____

Class: _____ **Semester:** _____

Number of Tardies: _____ **Number of Hours Absent:** _____

Objective	Very Satisfactory 3	Satisfactory 2	Unsatisfactory 1	Comments
Exhibits professional written communication (e.g., appearance, language, grammar)				
Uses the class materials appropriately (e.g., equipment, supplies, computers, cleanup)				
Provides instructor with all necessary information in a timely and organized manner (e.g., meets due dates, make-ups turned in within a week)				
Adheres to specific course policies (e.g., make-up guidelines, skill check-offs, externship guidelines)				
Projects a positive attitude and motivation (e.g., seen during lectures and labs)				
Displays professional verbal communication at all times (e.g., respectful, tactful)				
Maintains confidentiality of all personal interactions at all times (see rules of confidentiality in handbook)				
Projects professional work ethics (e.g., responsible, accountable, independent, full use of laboratory time: practice, study, computer)				
Cooperates with fellow students (e.g., team projects, skill practice, study groups)				
Displays responsible attendance behavior (e.g., arriving on time, calling in if detained or absent, prepared for next class session)				
Dresses appropriately (see handbook)				

Additional Comments: _____

_____

_____

Student Signature _____ **Instructor** _____

259

NOTE

NOTE